COMPLETE BOOK OF

Roasts, Boasts and Toasts

Elmer Pasta

Parker Publishing Company, Inc.
West Nyack, New York

© 1982, by

PARKER PUBLISHING COMPANY, INC.

West Nyack, N. Y.

Eighth Printing . . . . . July 1987

Library of Congress Cataloging in Publication Data

Pasta, Elmer,
    Complete book of roasts, boasts, and toasts.

    1. Public speaking—Handbooks, manuals, etc.
2. American wit and humor. 3. Occupations—Quota-
tions, maxims, etc. 4. Toasts. I. Title.
PN4193.I5P34   818'.5402   82-6296
ISBN 0-13-158329-8   AACR2

Preface

"During my two-plus decades in Hollywood, I suppose I have taken part in at least 1,000 Roasts, Boasts or Toasts of one sort or another.

At best, being the emcee, roaster or roastee makes one affably befuddled if you are not prepared or do not have the material that makes those zingers become electric.

Elmer Pasta, a talented writer and registered silly twirp (whom I first met when he was getting his BA in Journalism), has put in many hours of snorkling in his gag files to bring you this tome.

I wish that I had such a volume when I began doing whatever it is I do.

Elmer is an outstanding gentleman except for those rare occasions when he sets his nostril hairs on fire."

... Gary Owens
Supreme High Nurgle
Golden West Broadcasters
Hollywood, California

(Former "Laugh-In" regular and veteran Los Angeles d.j.)

What This Book Will Do for You

ROASTS   Do you know a fat, balding accountant with a big nose, who is also cheap and plays a bad game of golf? How about a blond, bombshell waitress with a fantastic figure, who likes to gossip and bet on the ponies?

Both these people, although quite different from each other, probably actually exist someplace. But even if you don't know these folks personally, you will find this book's list of Roasts vital in composing a funny speech (also popularly known as a roast) to fit just about anybody.

Here's a categorized guide of specific gags in several common areas that point out the distinctive characteristics or oddities of numerous individuals. When these jokes are appropriately combined, you have all the material for a humorously stylized, "custom" roast for any friend, relative or foe.

You can deliver an entire humorous routine aimed at a specific person, cleverly placing sharp zingers that emphasize all of his or her personality quirks. The jokes, of course, are made all the funnier because they often contain that familiar "grain of truth."

Put people in their place. Make fun of them without hurting their feelings or getting yourself punched out. Cover all the basic elements of a person—his or her profession, hobbies, personality and physical traits—humorously in one speech.

BOASTS   If you are the honoree, or victim, of a roast you will need this book's many Boasts that are in the same categories as the Roasts. Use them to come back at your tormentors. You will be well prepared to give clever answers to any humorous slights put upon you. Won't they be surprised!

Put insulters in their place. Be envied for coming out on top. Show them you can "dish it out" as well as take it.

TOASTS   There's always time to lift a glass in tribute to the honored guest. This book's many Toasts, also listed in the same categories as the Roasts and Boasts, sum up the character of the person roasted and usually conclude the program. They let everyone know that the joking was really meant in good fun, and the roast was just in jest.

THE TOTAL ROAST   Sectioned and alphabetized for easy use, this book contains nearly 3,000 sizzling gags for over 400 different professions, almost 100 hobbies, over a dozen relatives and friends, and more than 50 personalities and physical traits.

    Not only is this book helpful as a working tool, it also provides entertaining reading in itself.

A LITTLE ROAST HISTORY   The roast—a good-natured but mostly caustic, humorous tribute to a popular person or loved one—has been around for a long time. The super-insult speech, pointed at a particular victim, began at dinner meetings of men's clubs and fraternal lodges. They remain a familiar social event today, especially in entertainment organizations like the well-known Lamb's Club, Masquer's Club and Friar's Club.

    The roast has become even more popular through television. The "Dean Martin Celebrity Roast" and other network personality tributes, are consistently tops in the ratings. There was also a Broadway play titled "The Roast."

    This revived interest in the roast has increased the number of these types of speeches in everyday use. All kinds of local clubs for both men and women are having roasts of their members. Roasts are also as popular as ever now at gatherings of friends and relatives at birthday, anniversary and retirement fetes.

    Yes, the roast is now bigger than ever, obviously a hit at many a party. With insult comics like Don Rickles and Rip Taylor appearing on TV and in nightclubs regularly, the roast is surely here to stay.

HOW TO USE THIS HANDBOOK   Let's say you've decided to roast a friend or relative at an upcoming event. First, list everything you know about the person—his or her profession, hobbies, marital status, personality quirks and physical traits. Then, just look up each fact you've listed under the appropriate categories in this book. You've got all the makings of a roast right here—just put them all together.

Say you've been forewarned that you will be the subject of a roast. List all your own personal characteristics and look them up here. Jot down the Boasts under each category. You will be ready to deflect all those arrows with outrageous wit.

Also, if you are called upon or feel moved to toast the guest on some occasion, this handbook is the perfect guide for that. Just look up Toasts under each category.

You will notice that almost all the gags in this book alternate between male and female subjects. This is to add variety to the text and to demonstrate that either sex can be made the point of a joke.

Some professions are other people's hobbies or vice versa. So, be sure to look up both categories for material. Many jobs have different titles, i. e., attorney/lawyer. So, if you don't find a particular vocation right away, check under alternate possibilities.

By cross-checking the categories, you will see that many jokes can be easily adapted to fit other listings under the same topic. For example: under "Guitar Player," the line, "He's been having trouble with his guitar lately—people keep hitting him over his head with it!" could also be used to rib a violinist by substituting the proper musical instrument. The same joke is again useable for a tennis player by saying, "He's been having trouble with his tennis racquet lately— his opponents keep hitting him over his head with it!" Just use your imagination.

The same idea is possible, with some easy word switching, to turn many of the Roasts and Boasts into appropriate Toasts, or the Boasts into Roasts or Toasts, etc. Many variations of the same jokes may be written in the "Hobbies" category as with tennis and golf, by merely changing the type of ball.

By using this handbook and a little basic ingenuity you will come off as a very funny person. The jokes might even allow you to blow off some steam against someone while letting you look good. Always keep in mind, however, whether it's Roasts, Boasts or Toasts— have fun!

Table of Contents

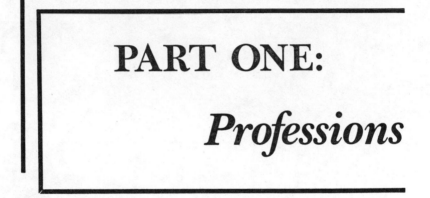

PART ONE:

Professions

A

ACCOUNTANT

ROASTS   He's an accountant—on account of he couldn't find a job doing anything else!

She must really be some accountant—her husband has to balance the family checkbook!

The real accounting comes after a night on the town with the boys—to his wife!

Just look at the clothes she's wearing tonight! She may be an accountant, but there's no accounting for taste!

BOAST   My boss says I'm a responsible accountant. If anything goes wrong at the office—I'm responsible!

TOAST   I toast the accountant! Everyone knows what an accountant is—he's the guy who tells you what to do with your money, after you've done something else with it!

ACROBAT

ROASTS   He's a true acrobat—when he first met his wife, he just flipped over her!

When they asked her if she wanted to be an acrobat, she said she'd give it a tumble!

He became an acrobat quite naturally—he was born a bouncing baby boy!

She has a trade secret for being a successful acrobat—Mexican Jumping Beans!

BOAST   I combine being a great acrobat along with being a true friend. I'll bend over backward for you!

TOAST   Here's a toast to a gal who all the guys think is a great acrobat—they like to jump on her!

ACTOR /ACTRESS

ROASTS   She's always talking about her last movie or her next husband!

I wouldn't want to imply he's lost his looks, but he's the only actor who could play the Frankenstein monster without makeup!

She gets a lot of terrific parts because she uses all her terrific parts to get them!

He recently made two legendary pictures at the same time—his first and his last!

BOAST   I worked all my life to be well-known. Now I have to wear dark glasses to avoid being recognized!

TOAST   Here's a toast to the poor stage actor. For him, it's curtains every night!

ACUPUNCTURIST

ROASTS   He became an acupuncturist quite naturally—his wife has been needling him for years!

As an acupuncturist she's constantly worried about her job—it has her on pins and needles!

He's a very enterprising acupuncturist—always trying to make points with his patients!

She's really no different than any other type doctor—always trying to stick it to her patients!

BOAST   I'm thinking of becoming an acupuncturist for disk jockeys by using phonograph needles!

TOAST   Here's a toast to a doctor of the ancient Chinese practice of acupuncture. It works well except that half an hour later, you have to see him again!

ADVERTISING PERSON

ROASTS   One of his biggest accounts is a new bourbon toothpaste. You get 90% more cavities but you don't give a damn!

It's amazing how she can give a favorable image to everything—everything but herself!

He's so dedicated to advertising that he wrote to his Congressman about too many highways defacing his billboards!

I wouldn't want to say her advertising copy lacks excitement, but her last commercial was sent live and arrived dead!

BOAST   I thought of a new slogan for the makers of penicillin: "The ideal gift for the person who has everything!"

TOAST   Here's a toast to an ad man who's got some hot ideas—too bad they're only half-baked!

AIR CONDITIONING PERSON

ROASTS   Because of him, you don't have to wait until winter to catch a cold—you can have one all year 'round!

She's so helpful in her job. Thanks to her, people can't work in the summer unless their teeth are chattering!

He really works cheaply. For a dollar and ninety-eight cents, he'll blow on an ice cube aimed at your face!

She's so loyal to her job she even has air conditioning in her compact—not her car, but her compact!

BOAST   I can do my job anywhere. Once I even air conditioned a steam room!

TOAST   Here's a toast to an expert on air conditioning—at least all the guys say she knows all about being frigid!

AIR FORCE PERSON

ROASTS   With his terrible flying reputation, he shouldn't be in the Air Force, he should be in the Air *Farce*!

She joined the Air Force because she knew she was no earthly good!

He joined the Air Force so he could learn to fly from the ground up!

She was a real candidate for the Air Force. She gets air-sick just licking an airmail stamp!

BOAST   I really have a lot of experience in flying—I fell out of a window once!

TOAST   Here's a toast to a true Air Force person—he gets dizzy when his barber pumps the chair too high!

AIR TRAFFIC CONTROLLER

ROASTS   She knows how risky it is to fly nowadays—she and her husband are so cautious, they take separate elevators!

He likes to date stewardesses built like his airport working conditions—well-stacked!

She's so dedicated to her job, she uses radar at night to get to the bathroom!

He knows how to direct a giant 747 to a terminal gate, yet he can't get his own car into a parking space!

BOAST   I'm so good at directing in pilots blind, the control panel on my board is in Braille!

TOAST   Here's a toast to a guy who is just great at directing air traffic into the terminal. Now if only he could find our luggage for us!

ANESTHESIOLOGIST

ROASTS   He's such a lazy anesthesiologist. He's the one who always falls asleep on the job!

She sincerely likes her job. In fact, she thinks it's a real gas!

He's so dictatorial in his profession—all of his patients have to take it lying down!

She may put you to sleep pretty good, but the real awakening comes when you receive her bill!

BOAST   I could also easily become a baseball umpire, because I'm an expert at telling when people are out!

TOAST   Here's a toast to an expert anesthesiologist—all he has to do is tell one of his long-winded jokes to put you to sleep!

ANIMATOR

ROASTS   At the slow speed her body moves, it's difficult to believe she's an animator!

He gets girls into his apartment by asking them to come up and see his animations!

She's some animator—her kid has to help her keep within the lines in a coloring book!

He came by his animator job quite naturally—his whole life is a cartoon!

BOAST   When somebody tells me, "See you in the funny papers," they really mean it!

TOAST   Let's lift a toast to a loyal animator. Every year, he takes the day off on Mickey Mouse's birthday!

ANNOUNCER

ROASTS   He's so terrible at his job, the most welcome thing he could announce is his retirement!

She started her job in an unusual way—announcing for captioned radio!

He just naturally has to get into radio announcing—he was too ugly to be seen on television!

The most startling thing she could ever announce would be her true age!

BOAST   I started my job at an early age. When I was born, I announced my own height and weight!

TOAST   Here's a toast to the announcer—like little children, he should be seen and not heard.

ANTIQUE DEALER

ROASTS   He specializes in selling a good antique—something no one would want if everyone had one, and everyone wants when no one has one!

There's one thing you should never say when entering her antique store—"What's new?"

He recently bought a genuine moustache cup. He claims it's genuine because it still has the moustache inside!

She's an antique dealer truly dedicated to her profession. She only eats junk food!

BOAST   I bought a genuine George Washington desk today. I know it's genuine, because it has Washington's name carved in the Formica!

TOAST   Here's a toast to the antique dealer. He knows one man's junk is another man's rare antique!

APARTMENT MANAGER

ROASTS   She said she has a lush apartment for rent. I believed her when I tripped over a drunk!

One tenant complained that his place was so small he couldn't afford a wife—he needed a wifette!

One of her apartments is so small, when you open the door you crack the mirror!

The walls in his apartments are so thin, when you peel onions the people next door cry!

BOAST   All my apartments have nice views but there's no overlooking the rent!

TOAST   Here's a toast to our apartment manager—the only way you can get her to paint your apartment is to move out!

APPLIANCE REPAIR PERSON

ROASTS   He repairs appliances all day long, but his wife can't get him to do as much as change a lightbulb!

Her own washing machine is so old, the paddles keep knocking her hat off!

His own oven is so old, he has to rub two sticks together to get it started!

She specializes in repairing stoves because she feels at home on the range!

BOAST   After I fix your washer, all your shirts will come out nice and white—even the green ones!

TOAST   Let's lift a toast to an appliance junkie—someone who's always in need of a good fix!

APPRAISER

ROASTS   He's so busy appraising, there's one thing he should really appraise—his marriage!

She appraised a house recently by saying it was without a flaw. Well, it didn't have much of a roof, either!

He's very subtle in his job. He recently appraised a car by concluding that if it were a horse it should be shot!

She appraised a house with rugs so thick, you needed snowshoes to get to the bathroom!

BOAST   I once appraised an antique table as going back to Louis XIV. Actually, it went back to Sears the next day!

TOAST   Here's a toast to an appraiser who obviously knows true value. What other reason would he have for wearing clothes like that?

ARCHEOLOGIST

ROASTS   He's trying to figure out how long people have been on earth while everybody else is worried about how much longer they'll be here!

She'll readily talk about the age of man, but she refuses to tell how old she is!

His claim to fame is discovery of the old Eskimo legend: "Don't eat the yellow snow!"

Her archeology professors advised her to become a bone specialist—they said she had the head for it!

BOAST   Isn't it just amazing? The older my subject gets, the younger I get!

TOAST   Here's a toast to a dedicated archeologist. He's the only man who made the city tear down six new blocks to make way for a slum!

ARCHITECT

ROASTS   She was thinking architecturally when she met her husband. Even then, she had designs on him!

Not everyone knows how he first became such a famous architect. He designed the golden arches for McDonalds!

She once designed a snowbank for Eskimos to keep their cold cash!

His job resembles his sex life—every time, it's back to the drawing board!

BOAST   I'm a very exacting architect. I even measure my clients before I design their breakfast nook!

TOAST   Let's lift a toast to a self-made architect. She's just lucky the building inspectors didn't come around during the construction!

ARMY PERSON

ROASTS   He was a war baby. His parents took one look at him and started fighting!

She has a heart like the U.S. Army—open to all men between the ages of 18 and 35!

He's an Army person now, but was something else in civilian life— happy!

As an Army wife, she used to send her overseas husband nagging letters. He couldn't even enjoy the war in peace!

BOAST   I really enjoyed living in an Army tent. At least I had no room to complain!

TOAST   Here's a toast to a really dedicated Army person—his license plates read, "HUP 2-3-4!"

ARTIST

ROASTS   He thought his first wife was as pretty as a picture, so he hung her!

She used to date another painter but he kept giving her the brush!

He wanted to do his mother-in-law in oil but he couldn't find a big enough vat!

The only thing she can draw successfully is a roomful of flies!

BOAST   I'm a very courageous painter—I sign my name to my paintings!

TOAST   Let's lift a toast to an artist who just completed a beautiful painting—and he didn't miss any of the numbers!

ASSEMBLER

ROASTS   She's so dumb, she has trouble assembling a complete thought!

He's so dumb, he has trouble assembling his kid's bike at Christmas!

The only part of her work title that fits her character is the first three letters.

He works like he was part of the committee who put the camel together!

BOAST   I'm so terrific at my job, the city has asked me to run for assemblyman!

TOAST   Here's a toast to a sex-shy assembler—her parts are hard to get!

ASTROLOGER

ROASTS   She was born under the sign of the lion—her mother was at an MGM movie at the time!

He's so empty-headed he was born under the sign "Vacancy!"

Her mother had so many children, she wanted the last one born under the sign "Stop!"

He may be an astrologer, but he hasn't had a sign of intelligence for years!

BOAST   I know the planets rule men's lives, but the men say that it's their wives!

TOAST   Here's a toast to a true astrologer—he lures girls to his apartment to show them their charts!

ASTRONAUT

ROASTS   He found out that athletes have athlete's foot, and that astronauts have missile toe!

She brags that space people are required to have high intelligence. But nobody likes a smart astronaut!

He's such a dumb astronaut, on his last flight he forgot where he was and called for a stewardess!

She says the space program is worthwhile. It's just a good thing we're not paying her by the mile!

BOAST   I really like my job as an astronaut. But just once, I'd love to ride with the top down!

TOAST   Let's lift a toast to an astronaut with true nerve—the first person to moon the Man-in-the-Moon!

ASTRONOMER

ROASTS   He can predict an eclipse of the sun years in advance, but can't forecast the weather over the weekend!

She's an astronomer quite naturally—because she's so spaced!

He's still trying to figure out why he sent a message to Mars and got a busy signal!

She helped discover what's on the dark side of the moon—people who don't pay their electric bills!

BOAST   You can obviously tell I'm an astronomer—I have such a heavenly body!

TOAST   Here's a toast to a dedicated astronomer—he drives a Mercury and only eats Mars bars!

ATTORNEY

ROASTS   Her court presentations are like a dice game—a lot of crap!

He wanted to be a lawyer for a nudist colony but they don't allow suits there!

She doesn't encourage her clients to commit perjury in court. She does it for them!

You know he's a lawyer—whenever he sends his clothes to the laundry, he forgets his briefs!

BOAST   I'm such a great lawyer, once I got the jury so confused they sent the judge to jail!

TOAST   Let's lift a toast to a great lawyer. He knows it's often better to know the judge than to know the law!

AUCTIONEER

ROASTS   You can easily tell he's an auctioneer. He's a man of more-bid tastes!

She's a true auctioneer—she always looks forbidding when conducting sales!

He'll sell you nothing for something if you're looking for something for nothing!

She says her job is very tiring, but she does see a lot of auction!

BOAST   Certainly I'm a great auctioneer—I don't give a rap for nothing!

TOAST   Here's a toast to the auctioneer—the one man you should never lift a hand to!

AUTHOR

ROASTS   He deserves to be a highly-paid writer—he also has to read the stuff while he's writing it!

She claims to reach millions of readers. It's a good thing they can't reach her!

His book is so bad, it must have been written on a tripe-writer!

She writes almost every day—home, for money!

BOAST   I sold everything during my writing career. I sold my car, my watch, my dog—everything!

TOAST   Let's raise a toast to the author—someone who has to pay an educated secretary to straighten out his mangled sentences!

AUTO DEALER

ROASTS   He was destined to become an auto dealer—his ancestors were horse thieves!

She sells a car that could become a real collector's item—it was made entirely in America!

The cars he sells are made for three people—one drives and two push!

She was trying to get a new car for her husband but nobody would trade!

BOAST   I've come up with a new dashboard item for cars. It's a little sign that pops up each date a payment is due!

TOAST   Let's toast the used car dealer—with him, it's difficult to drive a bargain!

B

BABY-SITTER

ROASTS   We worry about our baby-sitter's experience with kids. She says she knows the ropes!

He's such an absent-minded baby-sitter, he puts the TV to bed and watches the baby!

Now that all the kids have electric blankets, she doesn't tuck them in, she *plugs* them in!

He likes the kids to share everything with the baby-sitter, but not the mumps, measles or chicken pox!

BOAST   I have a terrific idea on how baby-sitters could make a fortune—giving tired blood transfusions to over-active kids!

TOAST   Here's a toast to a fine baby-sitter but sometimes she has to really restrain herself from sitting on the kids!

BAIL BONDS PERSON

ROASTS   He's known as "Old Man River"—always singing, "Tote that barge, lift that bail!"

She's so terrible in her job she couldn't bail out a sinking rowboat!

One of his clients went to jail for something he didn't do—pay his taxes!

One of her clients went to jail for stabbing his wife 62 times. He couldn't turn off the electric knife!

BOAST   All my clients are very obliging. They don't mind being interrupted in mid-sentence!

TOAST   Let's lift a toast to a fine bail person—someone who proves everyday that crime *does* pay!

BAKER

ROASTS   He likes being a baker. It keeps him rolling in dough!

She tried baking a birthday cake but the candles kept melting in the oven!

He's so terrible at his job, everything he does comes out half-baked!

She quite naturally is a baker—she certainly has the crust for it!

BOAST   I like being a baker—it's the only job in which you get paid to loaf!

TOAST   Here's a toast to a fine baker—he's a real friend in knead!

BANKER

ROASTS   I wouldn't want to say his financial situation is bad, but last night he broke open his kid's piggy bank!

They've been having so many holdups at her bank, they just installed revolving doors for the bandits!

He has a hard time getting all his vice-presidents to attend a directors' meeting—the public always thinks there's a run on the bank!

You can tell she's a banker—her customers give her withdrawal pains!

BOAST   My bank will gladly lend you money, provided you can prove you're already so well off you really don't need it!

TOAST   Here's a toast to a woman who's a true banker—all the guys have a lot of interest in her!

BARBER

ROASTS   Whether he's shaving your face or telling you old stories, he's always cutting up!

She's always confused when she gives another barber a haircut. Which one does the talking?

He charges so much for a haircut, he's really running a clip joint!

She probably doesn't recognize me from the last time I visited her shop—my face is all healed up now!

BOAST   For each of you here tonight, I'll charge only four dollars per haircut. That's one dollar for each corner of your head!

TOAST   Let's lift a toast to a fine barber—a man you always have to take your hat off to!

BARTENDER

ROASTS   He's such a dumb bartender, if you ask him for a stiff drink, he puts concrete in it!

She likes to mix her special "Factory Whistle" drink: one blast and you're through for the day!

I asked him for something tall, cool and full of booze—he brought out his wife!

She expects a 50-cent tip on a two-dollar check for a 35-cent bottle of beer!

BOAST   I once worked a bar with three bartenders—two for mixing drinks and one for listening!

TOAST   Let's lift a toast to a true bartender—a person to whom almost everything is a stirring event!

BEEKEEPER

ROASTS   He's obviously a beekeeper, that's why he calls all the girls "Honey!"

She claims to know the intelligence of bees. At least she always gets their point!

You know he's a beekeeper because he always has hives!

You know she's a beekeeper—her all-time favorite movie is "The Sting!"

BOAST   My insects are of extremely high intelligence. They're *spelling* bees!

TOAST Here's a toast to a true beekeeper—his favorite drink is a stinger!

BELLPERSON

ROASTS You can easily tell he's a bellboy because he's such a ding-a-ling!

She's so dumb, a guest asked her to bring him a deck of cards and she made fifty-two trips!

He's so terrible at his job, he's the only bellboy who brings warm icewater!

She's so particular a bell person, she won't take your laundry to be cleaned unless you wash it first!

BOAST I'm such a great bellman, when I finally leave my job they should retire my clanger!

TOAST Here's a toast to a terrific bellperson—someone who has a constant ringing in his ears!

BILL COLLECTOR

ROASTS He may be great at collecting other people's bills but he never pays any himself!

The people who have trouble meeting bills never seem to have any trouble dodging her!

His wife is also a bill collector—she collects tens, twenties, fifties and hundreds!

When she had a baby she sent it a bill because it was overdue!

BOAST   I'm so good at my job, I bring in more bills than a Congressman!

TOAST   Here's a toast to a stubborn bill collector, he won't give anybody credit!

BIOLOGIST

ROASTS   She may be an excellent biologist, but her own life couldn't bear up under a microscope!

He crossed a ferocious lion with a parrot. He doesn't know what he got, but when it talks, he listens!

She knows the true worth of a man, about a dollar ninety-eight!

He discovered why the dogs in Siberia are the fastest in the world—the trees are so far apart!

BOAST   I'm working on a great idea—crossing Limburger cheese with Chlorophyll!

TOAST   Let's lift a toast to a biologist who claims to know a lot about man. . . now if he could only figure out women!

BLACKSMITH

ROASTS   He started his job slowly, making little, tiny shoes for horseflies!

She's a dedicated blacksmith. Her favorite song is "The Anvil Chorus!"

He's a true blacksmith, all right—a man with a lot of horse scents!

She has no problems in her work because she keeps on hammering them out!

BOAST   At least, if you bring me your horse to be shod, I never suggest a dozen other things that need fixing!

TOAST   Here's a toast to a great blacksmith—a person who is truly a skilled forger!

BODYGUARD

ROASTS   With the shape he's in, nobody will ever need to guard *his* body!

She's always well prepared on the job—she uses Right Guard deodorant!

He just got a really big assignment, guarding a student body!

She may be good at guarding a body, but she's terrible at guarding body odor!

BOAST   I constantly have to guard my own body—so many women keep flinging themselves against it!

TOAST   Let's lift a toast to a person who likes to watch bodies, something many of us do for nothing!

BODY REPAIR PERSON

ROASTS   He takes such good care of other people's bodies it's too bad that he doesn't do something about his own!

She's an expert at her work because she knows all about being dense!

He's very successful working in body repair. He always does a bang-up job!

She deals daily with very sick cars—they all have the bends!

BOAST   I get my work done well. I always insist on hammering things out!

TOAST   Here's a toast to a man who really knows his job. He's a fender mender for the fender bender!

BOOKKEEPER

ROASTS   She's a real bookkeeper, all right—she steals them from the public library!

He calls himself a bookkeeper, but everyone else knows he's really a bookie!

You can tell she's a bookkeeper, even her apartment has a double entry!

He gets most of his daily exercise by running up his columns!

BOAST   I'm a great bookkeeper—I never let anybody borrow any!

TOAST   Here's a toast to a true bookkeeper—a person who feels good when things start looking black again!

BOOKIE

ROASTS   He once booked bets on a race for three-year-olds. It's disgusting what some parents will do for money.

As a true bookie, she knows that the best way to stop a runaway horse is to bet on it!

If you don't pay your losses with him, it's "You Bet Your Life!"

With her, money talks, but it doesn't say when it's coming back!

BOAST   I once had a 9 to 5 job in Las Vegas. It wasn't a very good job, but I liked the odds!

TOAST   Here's a toast to a true bookmaker—a pickpocket who lets you use your own hands!

BOTANIST

ROASTS   She's obviously a botanist—she grows wild in the woods!

He discovered why flowers are so lazy—most of them are in beds!

She looks like she's into plants. . . she's always potted!

His interests are similar to a politician's—they're both into graft!

BOAST   I don't understand why I'm being sued over the title of my new plant book. It's called "Roots!"

TOAST   Let's lift a toast to a great botanist—a person who is always a budding success!

BOTTLER

ROASTS   At the end of a hard day, he suffers from *bottle* fatigue!

She has a lot of jokes from her job. . . at least she says she knows quite a few corkers!

He treats his girl friends like bottles. He returns them after they've been used!

She always has her mind on the job—she thinks Beethoven's Fifth is a bottle!

BOAST   I'm truly dedicated to my job. My favorite song is "The *Bottle* Hymn of the Republic!"

TOAST   Here's a toast to a person truly dedicated to his job— he has no respect for age unless its bottled!

BOXER

ROASTS   Some say he's the best fighter in the country. But, he always gets beaten in the city!

She always orders the prize fighter's drink—punch!

He's known as the Rembrandt of boxing because he's so fond of the canvas!

She got into boxing for only one reason—she always wanted a striking affair!

BOAST   I'm a very prosperous boxer—I make money hand over fist!

TOAST   Let's lift a toast to a truly fine boxer, a man who always puts his best fist forward!

BREWER

ROASTS She also has a boyfriend who's a brewer. She really has the *hops* for him!

He had to take a special test to become a brewer, and he just *barley* passed it!

She even has beer in her waterbed—it's the only bed with a head!

He's really dedicated to his job—his favorite singer is Teresa Brewer!

BOAST I can boast one thing about my job—I produce plenty of liquid assets!

TOAST Here's a toast to a true brewer—he can always beer up under misfortune!

BRICKLAYER

ROASTS A whole coop of chickens came over to watch when they heard she was going to lay bricks!

The only thing he's good at doing on his job is *gold* bricking!

Some brick layer she is! Her house has a roll-away barbecue and an imitation fireplace!

He's a dedicated mason. His favorite person in American history is Stonewall Jackson!

BOAST I'm anything but a trouble-maker because I'm always cementing things!

TOAST   Here's a toast to a dedicated mason—she even eats brick
cheese!

BROADCASTING EXECUTIVE

ROASTS   He's so terrible at his job because he's more interested
in *broads* than broadcasting!

She may complain about the bad quality of programming, but she
doesn't have to go broadcasting it!

He doesn't understand why the public watches the bad programs on
the other station—he wants them to watch his!

The entertainment value of her programs is really quite extensive.
It ranges from fair to maudlin!

BOAST   There's one big thing listening to radio will always
have over watching television—no eyestrain!

TOAST   Here's a toast to a broadcaster whose programs reach
millions of people—he's lucky they can't reach him!

BUDGET PLANNER

ROASTS   He's a very stubborn budget planner. When he decides
on a figure, he won't budge it!

She's good at designing a system of worrying before you spend
instead of afterwards!

He has a plan for saving in which the outcome of the income depends
on the outgo for the upkeep!

She has a great system for saving money on vacations. By the time
she's balanced the budget, it's too late to go anywhere!

BOAST   I just figured my own family budget perfectly. The money we owe is the same amount we spent!

TOAST   Here's a toast to a real budget planner—he tells your money where to go instead of telling you where it went!

BUILDER

ROASTS   He's a great builder, all right, a builder of lies about how well he's doing!

There's one thing in particular she builds best—bills!

He should devote time to something that really needs building—like his body!

She's very interested in building. Right now, she's building up to a nervous breakdown!

BOAST   I came by my profession quite naturally because people are always building compliments about me!

TOAST   Here's a toast to a great builder—it's too bad his friends keep tearing him down!

BUS DRIVER

ROASTS   His bus sometimes gets so overcrowded, even he is left standing!

Her passengers often become so unruly, they ask *her* to step to the rear of the bus!

He used to drive a Greyhound but it insisted on stopping at every corner!

She only became a driver out of desperation, so she could get a seat on the bus!

BOAST   I really enjoy my job as a bus driver. I like telling people where to get off!

TOAST   Let's lift a toast to a bus driver who insists on never leaving on time—it would upset the schedule!

BUSINESS MANAGER

ROASTS   She's very good at managing other people's business, but she never manages to mind her own!

He's an excellent business manager, if you can manage to keep his hand out of your pocket!

She's such a good business manager, she's paying installments on the car she swapped for the car she traded in as part payment on the car she now owns!

As a business manager, he knows there's one sure way to make a client worry—tell him not to!

BOAST   Naturally, I'm good at managing other people's businesses—I'm so terrific at managing my own!

TOAST   Let's toast a great business manager—he spends time managing money for people, then manages to spend money killing time!

BUSINESS PERSON

ROASTS   He's always worried about the business outlook instead of being on the outlook for business!

Her business is fundamentally sound. . . asleep!

He's a true business man. He talks golf all morning at the office and business all afternoon on the links!

She's really at home in the business world, the place where it's always darkest before the merger!

BOAST   Business is so good, I don't have time to go to the bank to borrow the money to pay the rent!

TOAST   Here's a toast to a true business man—a guy who may be down, but he's never out of a conference!

BUTCHER

ROASTS   His meat prices are unbelievable today. It now costs an arm and a leg to buy some thighs and wings!

Some people think butchers make good money, but she has to do a lot of scrimping to make ends meat!

He cuts up such big pieces of meat, he's always doing business on a large scale!

She's a successful butcher because she's always taking short cuts to wealth!

BOAST   Everybody thinks I'm a funny butcher because I'm always cutting up!

TOAST   Let's lift a toast to a guy who really likes being a butcher because he can give people lots of tongue!

BUTLER

ROASTS   If he's lucky, he may live long enough to serve his third degeneration!

A butler is most often neither black or white—he was hired green!

Just like in the movies, if anything in the house is stolen, you can bet the butler did it!

You can easily tell he's a butler, he only does doors!

BOAST   I'm so loyal to my job, my favorite movie character is Rhett Butler!

TOAST   Here's a toast to a great butler—proof that they also serve who only stand and wait!

BUYER

ROASTS   Even as a mere child, her favorite repeated phrase was "Bye-bye!"

He's so terrible in his job the only thing he can buy is time!

She once bought a warehouse full of a million old calendars. She says if 1938 ever comes back, she'll be filthy rich!

He can't win a girl with traditional charm and wit—he has to buy 'er!

BOAST   I follow the motto, "If at first you don't succeed, buy, buy again!"

TOAST   Let's lift a toast to a terrific buyer—something even money can't buy!

C

CADDY

ROASTS   He can walk ten miles a day carrying heavy golf bags, but at home he has his kid bring him the ashtray!

She discovered something that will take ten points off any golfer's game—an eraser!

There are three big reasons why carts are better than caddies. They don't cost, they don't criticize and they don't count!

He's so disliked on the course, you don't know whether to call him a caddy or a cad!

BOAST   I'm very strict at scoring players. One golfer I was caddying had a stroke and I made him count it!

TOAST   Let's lift a toast to the faithful caddy—one of those little things that count!

CAKE DECORATOR

ROASTS   There are many people who are terrible at their jobs but she really takes the cake!

He's so bad at decorating cakes, his job is really going down the tubes!

She once messed up a cake so badly, they had to call in a re-decorator!

He may be good at decorating cakes, all right, but you should see what he did to his apartment!

BOAST   My decorating work is so beautiful, people sometimes eat the cake and save the frosting!

TOAST   Here's a toast to a true cake decorator—whenever you look at him he's always frosted!

CALLIGRAPHER

ROASTS   He has a lot of friends in the same business. They're all pen pals!

She had to take up calligraphy because she doesn't know how to type!

When time came to choose a likely profession, he saw the handwriting on the wall!

I'm not sure how good a calligrapher she is. Her favorite movie is "American Graffiti!"

BOAST   Good penmanship is something I just came by because of natural *ink*-stinct!

TOAST   Let's lift a toast to a great calligrapher—a person of many letters!

CAMP COUNSELOR

ROASTS   The only ones who appreciate camping with him are the mosquitoes.

With her camp cooking, it's just one canned thing after another!

His equipment is so old and outdated, camping with him is real camp!

She likes sending letters home from camp—begging for someone to get her out!

BOAST   The kids really like listening to my camp stories—they know they can't turn the dial!

TOAST   Here's a toast to counselor who really likes camping. That's why he's always in-tents!

CANDLESTICK MAKER

ROASTS   You can tell she's a candlestick maker because she only works *wick* ends!

He's obviously a candlestick maker because he's such a real dip!

She's so loyal to her job, she always wraps all her presents in wax paper!

He's so fond of his job, in his spare time he likes to wax the floors!

BOAST   I'm so good at my job, nobody can hold a candle to me!

TOAST   Let's lift a toast to a true candlestick maker. Even when mad, he'll wax indignant!

CARNIVAL WORKER

ROASTS   He should be used to working in a carnival—his home looks like a funhouse!

Obviously, she's a carnival worker because she always lets her best side show!

You can easily tell how he became a carnival worker—by *freak* accident!

She met her husband on a carnival Ferris wheel, and she's been taking him for a ride ever since!

BOAST   As a long-time carnival worker, my advice is: never take a check from the Indian Rubberman—they always bounce!

TOAST   Let's lift a toast to a carnival worker with a heavy problem—he's in love with the fat lady!

CARPENTER

ROASTS   He's obviously a carpenter, every thought to him has to be hammered across!

She's a very practical carpenter working on a house for room and board!

He's a terrible carpenter. He's always getting nailed by his boss!

She has a lot of fun on the job always saw-horsing around!

BOAST   I know I'm a great carpenter because I always measure up to the job!

TOAST   Here's a toast to a true carpenter—a person born to rule!

CARPET LAYER

ROASTS   He was once followed to work by a coop of chickens. They heard he was going to lay a rug and wanted to see how he did it!

She's so terrible at her job—she's always being called on the carpet!

If you hear from anyone that he's a good carpet layer, remember, there's not a *fiber* of truth to it!

She's so dumb, she cut a hole in her carpet so she could have a floor show!

BOAST   I know I'm a great carpet layer because I really know how to cut a rug!

TOAST   Let's lift a toast to a carpet layer who knows all about rugs. He used to be in the toupee business!

CARTOGRAPHER

ROASTS   She's such a terrible cartographer, she has to follow a map to get to the bathroom!

His mother started his interest early in life by always wrapping his school lunch in a roadmap!

She's so involved in her work, she even has her sex life charted!

He lost his first job some time ago when they had him stop giving out free maps at the gas stations!

BOAST   My maps sell big in Hollywood—drunken movie stars have to find their way home!

TOAST   Let's lift a toast to a fine map-maker—if only now he could show us how to re-fold them!

CASHIER

ROASTS   He calls himself a cashier but his work doesn't amount to anything!

She may work as a cashier, but she's so dumb nothing registers!

He's such a dumb cashier, everything in his brain registers "No Sale!"

She's such a dumb cashier, she thinks she should short-change all midgets!

BOAST   There's one good thing I can say about being a cashier—the job brings in a lot of money!

TOAST   Let's lift a toast to someone who works with a very popular musical instrument—the cash register!

CATERER

ROASTS   The guests at her last catered affair were speechless—they all died!

He once catered a group surgeon's dinner. He only served cold cuts!

She should certainly be a caterer, she knows all about having affairs!

You can tell he's a caterer. Everything his family eats at home are leftovers from parties!

BOAST   If everyone catered to their husband or wife as well as I do my clients there'd be a lot more happy marriages!

TOAST   Here's a toast to a person who specializes in serving catered food—something that's pretty hard to swallow!

CHARITY WORKER

ROASTS   He had to get into charity work because he quickly ran out of faith and hope!

She looks like a charity worker. All her clothes come from Goodwill!

He wanted to get into the Salvation Army to save bad girls but they wouldn't save him any!

She knows what real charity is: giving away what you can't use!

BOAST   I already collected over a million dollars for charity, and I haven't even found a disease for it yet!

TOAST   Here's a toast to a charity worker who has a tough job—raising money to stamp out telethons!

CHECKER

ROASTS   She may be a checker, but very little really registers with her!

He really has to work fast as a checker—the prices keep changing so quickly!

She's such an ugly checker, it only proves not all the bags are under the counter!

He's been checking food prices for years. As soon as they get cheaper, he might buy some!

BOAST   As a checker, I have a great idea for cutting your food bill in half—use a scissors!

TOAST   Let's lift a toast to a checker who always recommends a bargain—anything that's just slightly over-priced!

CHEF

ROASTS   His cooking is so bad even atheists pray before starting his meals!

She can turn your head with her looks and turn your stomach with her cooking!

The best way to lose weight is to try to eat his cooking!

If her electric can-opener ever blew a fuse, her customers would starve to death!

BOAST   I must say that my cooking is really improving. Now I've perfected my mashed potatoes to bite-size!

TOAST   Let's lift a toast to a great chef—it takes her two hours to cook Minute rice!

CHEMIST

ROASTS   Right now, she's working in chemical warfare—the eternal conflict between blondes and brunettes!

He's such a terrible chemist, he can't even mix a decent martini!

She likes to call ordinary things by such long names, you think she's talking about something else!

He's so dumb, he thinks the lab building is a chemical property!

BOAST   I really became a chemist quite naturally. I was a test-tube baby!

TOAST   Here's a toast to a not so successful chemist—everything he does goes down the tubes!

CHIMNEY SWEEP

ROASTS   Some folks wonder about him, he's always putting a damper on things!

Her job is the same every day—always looking black!

You can tell he's a chimney sweep, even his car goes "broom, broom!"

It's obvious she's a chimney sweep. Look how well-stacked she is!

BOAST   I'm a very independent chimney sweep. I only do things that soot myself!

TOAST   Let's lift a toast to an expert chimney sweep—we never have to worry about him falling down off the job!

CHIROPODIST

ROASTS   You can easily tell he's a chiropodist because he looks down at the heel!

She may be the attending chiropodist, but it's the poor patient who must *foot* the bill!

He was so dumb in college, for him to become a good chiropodist was quite a feets!

She's a chiropodist who, when given an inch, will always take a foot!

BOAST   I don't use an ambulance to bring injured patients to my office—I use a *toe* truck!

TOAST   Here's a toast to a fine chiropodist who's also a foot specialist—a true sole man!

CHIROPRACTOR

ROASTS   You have to feel sorry for her because she really has a back-breaking job!

He's really just like any kind of doctor, only interested in manipulating his patients!

She found out that becoming a chiropractor is expensive—you need a lot of backing!

He's a chiropractor who's also a coward because he's completely spineless!

BOAST   I just found a great place to open a new chiropractic office—right next door to a disco!

TOAST   Let's lift a toast to a fine chiropractor—a person whose fees are all *back* pay!

CHOREOGRAPHER

ROASTS   Even if he doesn't have his work ready on time, he'll always have a song and dance for you!

She's such a stubborn choreographer—she's only flexible from the neck down!

He developed his choreography technique in leaps and bounds!

She's not only light on her feet, but also light in her head!

BOAST   I just developed a terrific new dance step. All you do is tie your shoelaces together and disco!

TOAST   Here's a toast to a great choreographer—a person who is very handy with other people's feet!

CIRCUS PERFORMER

ROASTS   He started out as the class clown, but it was too much work putting on all that makeup every morning!

She became a tightrope walker because somebody told her it was a steady job!

He became a trapeze artist because he wanted to be a real swinger!

She naturally joined the circus because they wouldn't let her into Congress!

BOAST   I once joined the circus to be shot out of a cannon but I was fired! It wasn't my caliber job, anyway!

TOAST   Let's lift a toast to a performer who really started out working small—in a flea circus!

CLAIMS ADJUSTOR

ROASTS   She's such a terrible adjustor, she can't even settle a fight between her kids!

He's so crummy at his job, when he stands up he has trouble adjusting his shorts!

The only claim she could settle is that she doesn't have any brains!

He's so dumb, he couldn't settle a claim on an abandoned gold mine!

BOAST   I know I'm great at my job—even my psychiatrist says that I'm well-adjusted!

TOAST   Here's a toast to an adjustor who really wants to only claim one thing—attention!

CLERGY

ROASTS   Her sermons are so long, the congregation times them with a calendar instead of a clock!

As a clergyman, he finds it much easier to preach then to practice!

She's innoculated with a small dose of Christianity—enough to keep her from catching the real thing!

The preacher doesn't talk in his sleep, he talks in other people's sleep!

BOAST   Yes, I may look forward to the glorious wonders of heaven, but I'm in no great hurry to get there!

TOAST   Let's lift a toast to a great clergyman—someone who seems to think the eternal gospel requires an everlasting sermon!

CLERK

ROASTS   He's often called by another name that rhymes with his job title—and that name isn't Turk!

She's a billing clerk who had to go to a psychiatrist. She kept hearing strange invoices!

He's a file clerk who had to go to a psychiatrist. He found himself eating alphabet soup in the order A to Z!

She's a clerk who shares a staggered lunch hour at the office because everybody drinks!

BOAST   I know I'm a terrific clerk. I do all my work in permanent ink!

TOAST   Let's lift a toast to someone who long ago decided that a clerk must work—what an unpopular way of making money!

CLOTHIER

ROASTS   His work is no great achievement. He just lives off the *fad* of the land!

She lives off women who complain they have nothing to wear but who need several closets to keep it in!

He lives for fashion—something that goes in one year and out the other!

She makes sure her clothes go out of style as soon as they become fashionable!

BOAST   I owe my success to knowing the thing women's wear leaves to the imagination is what makes it so expensive!

TOAST   Here's a toast to a fine clothier—he knows fashion is as strange as its seams!

COAST GUARD PERSON

ROASTS   She should learn more about guarding our coasts against our greatest enemy—oil spills!

Everytime I call his house while he's on duty, his wife answers that the coast is clear!

She doesn't really patrol our nation's shores, she guards a roller coaster!

He was something very different before he joined the Coast Guard—happy!

BOAST   I love being in the Coast Guard. On a clear day when the fog lifts, you can see the smog in the city!

TOAST   Here's a toast to a really competent Coast Guard person—remember Pearl Harbor!

COCKTAIL WAITRESS

ROASTS   When guys at the bar ask for the specialty of the house—she's it!

She really got a great tip yesterday—don't go out with married men!

She's so dumb, during her break she goes to another bar to have a drink!

She puts olives in drinks for people who don't like to drink on an empty stomach!

BOAST   I may be just a cocktail waitress, but I always provide a lot of good spirits!

TOAST   Let's lift a toast to an enterprising cocktail waitress—she thinks money grows on *trays*!

COMEDIAN

ROASTS   He's such a terrible comic, he always gets a silent ovation!

She's so unfunny, she could silence a laughing hyena!

He's so unfunny, for him a solo appearance is overexposure!

You've heard of a stand-up comic—her audiences can't stand her lying down!

BOAST   I have a great memory for old jokes. I just hope nobody else does!

TOAST   Let's lift a toast to a true comedian—a person who has nerves to steal!

COMMUNICATIONS SPECIALIST

ROASTS   He calls himself a specialist, but he has trouble communicating with his wife and family!

Some communications specialist she is. She can't even use a telephone without misdialing!

He can't even communicate to a waiter what he wants for lunch!

You can tell she's a communications specialist—she puts all her boy friends on hold!

BOAST   My mother was also a communications specialist—she could talk on the telephone for hours!

TOAST   Here's a toast to a communications specialist who believes in getting back to basics—two Dixie cups and a string!

COMPUTER OPERATOR

ROASTS   She's such an ugly computer operator, men want to fold, bend and mutilate her!

If you want to give him a bad time, just mail back your computer bill cards with some extra holes punched in them!

She watches TV like a computer operator—always changing the program!

He failed working at a computer-dating service. Nobody wanted to date a computer!

BOAST   As a computer operator, I work just like a boxer—always waiting to *key* punch!

TOAST   Let's lift a toast to a fine computer operator—someone who has never heard of the term "human error!"

CONDUCTOR

ROASTS   His father was also a conductor—ever since the day he was struck by lightning!

She may know how to conduct a band, but she should learn how to conduct herself!

His father was also a conductor—not orchestra, train!

She's such a terrible conductor, she often doesn't know her brass from a bass drum!

BOAST   As a conductor I often get audience requests—but my baton is way too long!

TOAST   Here's a toast to a great conductor—a person who often doesn't know how to compose himself!

CONSTRUCTION WORKER

ROASTS   He's so stubborn in his work, underneath his hard hat he has a hard head!

She likes to stick to construction work for one reason—it's so riveting!

He once worked on a building that was so high, you had to play a harp to qualify for the job!

She's so crazy about her work, she wraps her lunch in old blueprints!

BOAST   I learned one thing about construction work: no matter how conditions improve, you always start in the hole!

TOAST   Here's a toast to a fine construction worker—he keeps tearing down old buildings to build new slums!

CONSULTANT

ROASTS   The only thing she's good at consulting lately is her own horoscope!

He uses the most modern scientific procedures in his consulting—a crystal ball!

She calls herself a consultant, which really means she's unemployed!

He's so terrible in his work, he has to consult his wife about which tie to wear in the morning!

BOAST   The consulting advice I give costs nothing, unless you decide to act upon it!

TOAST   Let's lift a toast to a terrific consultant—someone whose main job is giving detailed explanations of things he knows nothing about!

CONTORTIONIST

ROASTS   He's a contortionist naturally, because he's always wrapped up in himself!

She must not be able to hold a job because she's always looking for a different position!

He has a terrible attitude toward life. He really should take a different posture!

Naturally, she's a contortionist. She's often beside herself!

BOAST   I'm a very helpful contortionist because I'm always bending over backward for people!

TOAST   Let's lift a toast to a typical contortionist—someone who leads a double life!

CONTROLLER

ROASTS   He may be good at his job, but after a few drinks he loses complete control!

She works in the office as a controller, but at home she has no power over the kids!

He's usually out of the office so much, he has to run things by remote control!

She helps keep company expenditures within limits, but you should see her own credit card statements!

BOAST   I may control things at the office, but at home the kids control the TV set!

TOAST   Let's lift a toast to a fine controller. If only he'd keep his hands off the company air conditioning dial!

CORONER

ROASTS   He doesn't have much of a medical background, but he saw every episode of "Quincy!"

She thinks she has a great sense of humor because she's such a cut-up at autopsies!

He really likes his job because so many people are dying to meet him!

She thinks a natural death nowadays is being killed by a car!

BOAST   The best part of my job is that none of the people I work with complain!

TOAST   Here's a toast to a fine coroner—someone many a driver approaches at over 55 miles-per-hour!

COSMETOLOGIST

ROASTS   She knows that any product she uses should have high face value!

With the prices he charges, a woman's face is *his* fortune!

The way she flatters her customers, beauty isn't only skin deep, it's skin dope!

He may know a lot about cosmetics, but he has yet to make up with his wife!

BOAST   I once made a woman look so beautiful, even her husband wanted to go out with her!

TOAST   Let's lift a toast to an up-to-date cosmetologist. He's always interested in the latest wrinkle!

COSTUMER

ROASTS   The outlandish dresses he comes up with are more *gone* than gown!

Actually, her selection of clothes is very becoming—becoming worn out!

The costumes he chooses are so loud, they have to come with a volume control!

Her selection of costumes is just like her personality—loud!

BOAST   I'm really in my salad days as a costumer—excellent in my dressing!

TOAST   Let's lift a toast to a costumer who is very interested in clothes. It's too bad he's not interesting *in* them!

COURT REPORTER

ROASTS   She never goes to the beauty parlor for a permanent. She hears enough in court to curl her hair!

He thinks he leads a tough life—nothing but a daily series of trials!

When she's out of the courtroom, she's more jaw than law!

With his style of court reporting, he makes sure justice is dispensed . . . with!

BOAST   I enjoy working in law as a court reporter. It's my *in-laws* I can't stand!

TOAST   Here's a toast to a fine court reporter—a real witness to the persecution!

COWBOY/COWGIRL

ROASTS   He's good at roping in the daytime and ties one on pretty well at night!

She isn't really a very good cowgirl—she just likes to horse around!

He once worked a ranch with 30 thousand head of cattle—no bodies, just the heads!

She didn't really want to be a cowgirl—she was roped into it!

BOAST   Actually, I'm a terrific cowpuncher. Yesterday, I punched 60 cows!

TOAST   Here's a toast to a fine cowboy who sits tall in his saddle—from all his blisters!

CREDIT MANAGER

ROASTS   You have to really give her credit, since she won't give it to anybody else!

He may be called a Credit Manager by some people, but others have different names for him!

It's silly to call her a Credit Manager—she never manages to give any!

If you're interested in his letting you have a line of credit, you'd better have quite a line to get it!

BOAST   I'm always willing to give credit where credit is due. Unfortunately, it's never due anybody!

TOAST   Here's a toast to the Credit Manager—someone to whom we all owe a great deal!

CRIMINOLOGIST

ROASTS   He's so terrible at his job, all his work is a crime!

She knows there are too many crimes, but she can't say what the real number should be!

The detectives arrested him as a suspect, because he was always at the scene of the crime!

She never finds the criminal, unless he's unlucky enough to be caught!

BOAST   I've come to the conclusion that the only people who make housecalls these days are burglars!

TOAST   Here's a toast to someone who knows that crime doesn't pay, unless of course, you do it well!

CRITIC

ROASTS   Obviously, he's a critic because he loves to *hiss* and tell!

Obviously, she's a critic because she likes to go places and *boo* things!

You can easily tell he's a critic, because he's always down on thing
he's not up on!

She only writes because she has to say something—not because sh
has anything to say!

BOAST   Actually, it's easy to avoid criticism: say nothing
do nothing and be nothing!

TOAST   Let's lift a toast to a true critic—someone who like
to write about things he doesn't like!

CUTTER

ROASTS   You can easily tell what her job is because she's alway
making cutting remarks!

He originally learned his job in the military service as a Coast Guar
cutter!

She was fired from her last job. Instead of cutting, she was cuttin
up!

He got a ticket for doing his job in the car. He was cutting in and ou
of traffic!

BOAST   I can always get a good job as a cutter because I'm s
sharp!

TOAST   Let's lift a toast to a fine cutter—someone who neve
leads a dull life!

D

DAIRY WORKER

ROASTS   He knows one thing about a dairy worker's job: milk it for everything it's got!

She didn't come by her dairy worker job easily—she had to have a lot of pull!

He thinks cream costs more than milk because it's harder for the cows to sit on the smaller bottles!

She lost her last diary worker job because everything she did turned sour!

BOAST   I decided to become a dairy worker because I wanted to see the Milky Way!

TOAST   Here's a toast to a dedicated diary worker—someone who thinks his job is *udderly* fascinating!

DANCER

ROASTS   He claims he has dancing in his blood. Too bad it hasn't gotten to his feet yet!

She learned to disco very quickly when a waiter dropped an iced drink down her dress!

Dancers run in his family—too bad they don't dance!

She had to give up belly dancing because nobody could stomach watching her!

BOAST   I had to give up being a hula dancer—business was too shaky!

TOAST   Let's lift a toast to a gal who would make a great toe dancer—she dances on everybody's toes!

DELIVERY PERSON

ROASTS   He once wanted to be a boxer, but he couldn't deliver a punch!

She's a big come-on with the guys during a date, but when they get her home she won't deliver!

He likes dining on almost any part of a chicken but he won't eat de-liver!

She's so stuck-up, even her birth was a special delivery!

BOAST   Remember my slogan: "Don't let other people deliver your packages all broken. Hire *me* to do it!"

TOAST   Let's lift a toast to a delivery person who drinks on the job—someone who delivers everything smashed!

DEMOLITIONIST

ROASTS   She really has a demolitionist's personality—always exploding!

It's always dangerous being around him. You never know when he might blow up!

She's so insecure, if she ever lost her job she'd be demolished!

He's a natural for the job. He's so good at tearing down things!

BOAST   I'm so terrific at my job because I have such a dynamite personality!

TOAST   Here's a toast to a terrific demolitionist. Being around him is a real blast!

DENTIST

ROASTS   He was once married to a beautiful manicurist but they fought tooth and nail!

The only way she could be a painless dentist would be if she forgot to bill you!

His customers often complain a lot—whenever he gets on their nerves!

She had to become a dentist—what else was she going to do with all her old magazines?

BOAST   I tell jokes to my patients while I work. Sometimes I pull some pretty good ones!

TOAST   Let's lift a toast to a fine dentist who learned his profession in the army—as a drill sergeant!

DERMATOLOGIST

ROASTS   He can make your complexion look like a peach—yellow and fuzzy!

She can make your face look like a million—green and wrinkled!

He can make your face look like a movie star's—Lassie!

She won't treat your skin disease, unless you come up with enough scratch!

BOAST   Remember my motto: "Beauty is only skin deep, but ugly is rotten to the core!"

TOAST   Let's lift a toast to a dedicated dermatologist. His favorite hobby is skindiving!

DESIGNER

ROASTS   She's a designer who knows all the latest wrinkles in clothes—and shows it!

The only real designs he ever has are the ones he has on his secretary!

She comes up with hundreds of different designs. It's too bad they're all out of style!

His designs are so old-fashioned, he should draw plans for retirement!

BOAST   I'm such a perfect person—I wasn't just born, I was designed!

TOAST   Here's a toast to a great designer—a stylist who has *mode* in his eye!

DETECTIVE

ROASTS   She's such a terrible detective, the only thing she ever runs down are her heels!

He may sometimes get on the right track, but then he goes in the wrong direction!

She likes being a detective. The job allows her to get plenty of sleep!

The only reason he became a detective was because he likes sleeping in the open air!

BOAST   I'm not only a great detective, I also make a terrific barbecue. But then, I've always enjoyed a good steak out!

TOAST   Here's a toast to a fine detective—someone who found a great legal way of being dishonest!

DIAMOND CUTTER

ROASTS   He looks just like a diamond cutter—always stoned!

She's such a complainer, always griping about how rough things are!

His only previous experience as a diamond cutter was mowing the grass at Yankee Stadium!

She was fired from her last job as a diamond cutter and it was a shattering experience!

BOAST   They hired me as a diamond cutter for only one reason: because I'm such a gem!

TOAST   Let's lift a toast to a great diamond cutter—someone who has many facets to his job!

DIETICIAN

ROASTS   His idea of a proper diet is to eat less at the table and more between meals!

She thinks a proper diet is simply the triumph of mind over platter!

He says the right way to follow a diet is just to let the hips fall where they sway!

She gives all her patients mirrors so they can watch what they eat!

BOAST   I found out what a lot of my patients are allergic to—paying their bills!

TOAST   Let's lift a toast to a dietician who always gives his patients a complete checkup. They never live to regret it!

DIPLOMAT

ROASTS   She thinks a diplomat is something a diplo steps on when he gets out of the shower!

He's a true diplomat—long on protocol and very short on memory!

She's a natural diplomat. She lies a lot and somehow gets away with it!

He may sometimes lay his cards on the table, but he usually has another deck up his sleeve!

BOAST   I'm such a great diplomat, it seems like I'm always letting someone else have my way!

TOAST   Here's a toast to a great diplomat—he can convince someone he's a liar without actually telling him so!

DIRECTOR

ROASTS   The only thing he could direct is traffic, and then he'd probably jam it up!

She's some crazy director—she can't even have sex without giving directions!

He's such a terrible director, he can't even shave himself in the mirror without yelling, "Cut!"

She's such a lousy director, she can't even follow the directions on a box of cake mix!

BOAST   I really know my job well. Even when I seduce girls, I use the direct approach!

TOAST   Here's a toast to a true director—a man who enjoys his work, but the decisions are killing him!

DISH WASHER

ROASTS   She quit her last job because of depression. She was *dish*-illusioned!

He was fired because he was paying more attention to the dishes serving the food than the ones he had to wash!

She started working at a baseball stadium—washing home plate!

He quit his last job in despair. It wasn't all it was cracked up to be!

BOAST   I never wash dishes at home—people are always eating out of my hand!

TOAST   Here's a toast to a truly successful dish washer—someone who's had a lot of breaks!

DISC JOCKEY

ROASTS   You can easily tell he's a disc jockey—he lives on spins and needles!

She's a talkative disc jockey because she has the power of babble!

He's so annoying—he shouldn't be on the ether, he should be *under* it!

She's perfect for the job—she has a long-playing tongue!

BOAST   I put my record turntable in the refrigerator so I could play some cool music!

TOAST   Let's lift a toast to a great disc jockey—someone who was created to teach mankind the blessings of silence!

DISPATCHER

ROASTS   There's only one thing he doesn't dispatch at work—work!

She does such a terrible job, the only thing that really needs dispatching is her!

He's kept his job so long by keeping things so mixed up they don't dare fire him!

She doesn't dispatch slow and she doesn't dispatch fast—she dispatches half-fast!

BOAST   As a dispatcher, I say nothing is impossible—I've been doing nothing for years!

TOAST   Let's lift a toast to a terrific dispatcher—when it comes to work, he'll stop at nothing!

DITCH DIGGER

ROASTS   He's a natural ditch digger—everyone knows how good he is at shoveling it!

Many people call her by a name that rhymes with the thing she digs— and that name isn't witch!

He's so involved in his work, he calls his home his digs!

She may not get along too well with the women at work but the men really dig 'er!

BOAST   I'm really a great ditch digger because I'm so down to earth!

TOAST   Here's a toast to a terrific ditch digger—someone who is truly an ace in the hole!

DOCTOR

ROASTS   His medical practice is so good, he can't see another patient this year without going into a higher tax bracket!

She wanted to start as a baby doctor, but she couldn't reach the operating table!

He's a medical specialist—a nose, throat and wallet man!

She's a good doctor to go to if you want to reduce. After you see her, you won't have any money left to buy food!

BOAST   I'm one of the only doctors left who makes housecalls. Just let me know what time you can make it to my house!

TOAST   Here's a toast to a fine doctor—a man to whom we trust our lives and our fortunes!

DOG TRAINER

ROASTS   He used to have an army dog, but it wanted to be transferred to another post!

She claims that dogs from Siberia are the fastest in the world because the trees are so far apart!

He got a very nice dog for his wife. I wish I could make a trade like that!

Her dog is so afraid of burglars, she had to put an alarm system in the dog house!

BOAST   I call my dog "Spot." He's really all just one color, but you should see my rug!

TOAST   Here's to a man with a great doberman pincher. All day long, it goes around pinching dobermans!

DONUT MAKER

ROASTS   She's anxious to make a lot of money in her business because she's such a dough nut!

He invented a cracker donut for people who want to dunk their soup!

She was only a donut maker's daughter but she could take on a baker's dozen!

He invented a square donut to pack into lunch boxes!

BOAST   I'm such a generous donut maker—I charge nothing for the holes!

TOAST   Let's lift a toast to a safe donut maker—there's always a cop at his shop!

DOORPERSON

ROASTS   He's such an unlucky doorperson, yesterday he was arrested for loitering!

Naturally, she's a doorperson, she has quite a famous reputation as a swinger!

He's an opportunistic doorperson. He's always working on an opening!

She's worried about her job as a doorperson because it only hinges on one thing!

BOAST   I know when a door is not a door—when it's a jar!

TOAST   Let's lift a toast to someone who always gets things going at a party—because he's such a good opener!

DRAPERY INSTALLER

ROASTS   His job didn't come too easily—he had to have a lot of pull!

You can easily tell she's a drapery installer. At the end of the day she can hardly pull herself together!

He once was arrested for installing a curtain around a museum figure—the charge was statuary drape!

Her job is actually pretty easy—she spends most of her time just hanging around!

BOAST   I'm really sick and tired of getting the same old greeting: "How's it hanging?"

TOAST   Here's a toast to a great drapery installer—someone who knows if he doesn't do his job right, it's curtains!

DRIVER

ROASTS   I don't want to imply he's rough on a car, but for the first time in history, Ford has asked for its guarantee back!

She's been stopped so often by traffic cops, they finally gave her a season ticket!

He's really a very careful driver—he always slows down when going through a red light!

She bumped into some close friends yesterday. Naturally, she was driving!

BOAST   Listen, if you people don't like the way I drive, get off the sidewalk!

TOAST   Here's a toast to a terrific driver—he gets 25 miles to a fender!

DRIVING INSTRUCTOR

ROASTS   He's such a terrible instructor, he couldn't teach a carpenter how to drive a nail!

She's so terrible an instructor, she teaches her students to honk before they go through a red light!

You can easily tell he's a driving instructor because he's always horning in!

She's so dumb an instructor, she takes all her students out to the driving range!

BOAST   I'm a terrific driving instructor—I get over a thousand miles per student!

TOAST   Let's lift a toast to a great driving instructor—he knows that most auto accidents are caused by the nut behind the wheel!

DRY CLEANER

ROASTS   She drinks so much on the job, I don't see how she can call herself a dry cleaner!

He has a lot of kids working his place because he hates to see a grown man *dry*!

She charges so much, nowadays it's her customers who get taken to the cleaners!

He's done so much dry cleaning in his lifetime, he suffers from *clothes*-trophobia!

BOAST   I'm so overwhelmed with customers lately. I have a lot of pressing business!

TOAST   Here's a toast to a dry cleaner who guarantees the clothes he returns will never shrink—unless they get wet!

E

EDITOR

ROASTS   She edits copy just like she treats her friends—always cutting them!

As an editor, you might guess what his hobby is—he collects book ends!

She's concerned about editing as much as her sex life—always watching for periods!

He must be taking his editing job too seriously—his friends can read him like a book!

BOAST   My real ambition as an editor is to put a finishing touch to a story—a match!

TOAST   Let's lift a toast to an editor who reads so much, he gets asterisks in front of his eyes!

EFFICIENCY EXPERT

ROASTS   If she's such a great efficiency expert, how come she's never at work on time?

He should really become an earthquake expert—he's always finding fault!

She should really become a baseball announcer—she's so good at reporting errors!

The only reason he's an efficiency expert is because he doesn't have a business of his own to wreck!

BOAST   I could even improve the Ten Commandments—just cut them down to six or seven!

TOAST   Let's lift a toast to a great efficiency expert—someone who can figure out the time lost in every business but his own!

EGG CANDLER

ROASTS   He obviously has become the butt of every yolk!

She's so dedicated to her job that the only thing she grows in her garden is eggplant!

He must be very bored in his job. Every day he goes to work it's the same old shell game!

She really likes her job, but it's not all that it's cracked up to be!

BOAST   I know I'm terrific in my job—nobody else can hold a candle to me!

TOAST   Here's a toast to a great egg candler, even though he is a little hard-boiled!

ELECTRICIAN

ROASTS   He once knew a Navajo electrician who installed a light in his tribe's bathroom. He was the first Indian to wire a head for a reservation!

She became an electrician quite naturally—her father was a conductor!

He may be a good electrician, but his wife says he'll never see the light!

She may be the electrician, but it's the customer getting the bill who receives the shock!

BOAST   As an electrician, I read a lot of newspapers. I want to keep up on current events!

TOAST   Here's a toast to a very dedicated electrician—he's always putting in a good plug for his job!

ELECTROLOGIST

ROASTS   He had a hard time taking his electrologist test, but he passed it by a hair!

She's an expert electrologist—she's been needling people for years!

He didn't become an electrologist easily—he had to have a lot of pull!

She has to be patient with her customers. Many of them give her a lot of lip!

BOAST   People really enjoy my electrologist sessions—they seem to get a lot of charge out of them!

TOAST   Let's lift a toast to a fine electrologist—someone who believes in the motto, "Hair today, gone tomorrow!"

ELEVATOR OPERATOR

ROASTS   She really shouldn't complain, even though her job has a lot of ups and downs!

He quit his last job because his employers gave him the shaft!

She really likes her job. She keeps people up in the world!

There's one sure thing you can say about him, he's raised a lot of families!

BOAST   I really enjoy my job as an elevator operator—it always gives me a lift!

TOAST   Here's a toast to a fine elevator operator—the only person who makes a success of running other people down!

EMBALMER

ROASTS   He lost his last job because he couldn't get along with his boss—there was too much bad blood between them!

You can easily tell she's an embalmer—her favorite drink is a Bloody Mary!

You can easily tell he's an embalmer—his favorite breed of dog is the bloodhound!

As an embalmer, she makes special trips to the blood bank—to make withdrawals!

BOAST   I have a special name for my car—I call it my blood mobile!

TOAST   Here's a toast to a fine embalmer. In order to get his job, he had to take a blood test!

ENGINEER

ROAST   Her father was also a successful engineer. . . on the Southern Pacific Railroad!

She has fine hearing when it comes to listening to machines because she has such a good engine-ear!

He's so terrible at his job, he can't even engineer his car into a parking space!

As an engineer, she sits up all night worrying over things that a fool never even heard of!

BOAST   As an engineer, I'm quite a specialist—always called in at the last minute on a project so I can share the blame!

TOAST   Let's lift a toast to an ingenious engineer—a person always able to get others to do the work he dislikes!

ENGRAVER

ROASTS   He lost his last job because he misspelled a name on a tombstone and was "engrave" trouble!

She claims to be a skilled engraver. Others call her just a cheap chisler!

He calls himself an engraver because he doesn't want anybody to know he's really a mortician!

She's so fussy, an invitation from her to have sex comes engraved!

BOAST   I'm quite an educated engraver—everyone knows I'm a man of many letters!

TOAST   Here's a toast to a steadily working engraver—someone who's always got something lined up!

ENTERTAINER

ROASTS   She thinks she's such a great performer, but she couldn't even entertain a thought!

He's such a conceited entertainer that when he hears thunder he starts to take bows!

The only way she could get a standing ovation would be if she sang the "Star Spangled Banner!"

He's quite a promising entertainer—if only he'd promise to not entertain anymore!

BOAST   I once worked a night club where business was so bad, the waiters were dancing with the chairs!

TOAST   Let's lift a toast to a fine entertainer who works a lot for charity. She has to—nobody ever offers to pay her!

ENTOMOLOGIST

ROASTS   Naturally, he's an entomologist—because he likes to bug people!

She has plenty of experience as an entomologist—she used to plant bugs for the FBI!

Obviously, he's an entomologist—his favorite cartoon character is Bugs Bunny!

She's become so much like her insects, she has to wear a hat to cover her antennae!

BOAST   There's one thing good in my experience with entomology—people may bug me, but bugs never *people* me!

TOAST   Let's lift a toast to an enthusiastic entomologist—the only way to get rid of him is with bug spray!

ESTIMATOR

ROASTS   She's so terrible in her work, she can't even estimate how long she'll keep her job!

He's so terrible at his job, for him an estimate is usually a *guess*-timate!

She's so involved in her work, she can't even have sex without an estimated time of arousal!

He's so terrible at his job, he couldn't estimate the number of inches in a foot-long ruler!

BOAST   I'm the very best estimator there is. . . in everybody's estimation!

TOAST   Here' s a toast to a fine estimator with an open mind—it's always vacant!

EXERCISE INSTRUCTOR

ROASTS   The best exercise she could teach is running up bills!

The only exercise he could teach is jumping to conclusions!

She should teach *herself* to push away the second dinner plate at the table!

The only exercise he could teach is bending the truth!

BOAST   I'm so successful an exercise instructor because I have such a great student body!

TOAST   Let's lift a toast to an exercise instructor who isn't so great at helping you lose weight—just at rearranging it!

EXPLORER

ROASTS   He's already explored the entire world—now he wants to go someplace else!

She spends so much money on her job, her backers want to explore where it goes!

On his last trek, it took him six months to sing "Night and Day"—he was in Alaska at the time!

She never travels by plane—the long trip to the airport makes her car-sick!

BOAST   I never thought I'd come back alive from my last trip—I got caught at the lingerie counter in a department store sale!

TOAST   Let's lift a toast to a true explorer—he's still looking for big enough buns for an elephant ear sandwich!

EXPORTER

ROASTS   He tells people he's an exporter, but what he really means is that he used to be a railroad car attendant!

Her business is so shady, she's the only exporter to be *de*ported out of the country!

He calls himself an exporter, but he's really trying to unload surplus junk on foreigners at a profit!

She's so dumb, she's trying to export chopsticks to China!

BOAST   I'm such a great exporter, I just sold a million pair of snowshoes to Guam!

TOAST   Here's a toast to a colorful exporter—someone who knows what it is to go through a lot of red tape!

EXTERMINATOR

ROASTS   You can tell he's a determined exterminator, because he's always trying to get the bugs out of things!

She's obviously an exterminator, because she's such an expert at making a pest of herself!

Even as a little boy in school he knew his future calling because he was teacher's *pest*!

She's obviously an exterminator—her favorite cartoon character is *Bugs* Bunny!

BOAST   I really enjoy my work as an exterminator because often it's such a gas!

TOAST   Let's lift a toast to the exterminator's motto: let us *spray*!

F

FARMER

ROASTS   She's what you call a hula girl farmer—always rotating her crops!

He didn't make his cropland too big this year—his wife is starting to tire easily!

She put all her hens in a cement mixer so she could have scrambled eggs!

The farmhands all know what he really raises best—his temper!

BOAST   I like farming because I can pick up plenty of toma-
toes . . . and I don't have to whistle first!

TOAST   Let's lift a toast to a fine farmer—she learned that the
hardest part about farming is getting up at five a.m.!

FBI PERSON

ROASTS   With her, the letters F-B-I only mean one translation:
Friendly But Ignorant!

You can easily tell he works for the FBI—he likes to make a federal
case out of everything!

She's so terrible at her job, someone should investigate if she has
a brain!

He really belongs in the FBI—ever since he was a kid he's liked bugs!

BOAST   I once arrested a guy who was making big money—about
a quarter of an inch too big!

TOAST   Here's a toast to a sex-crazed FBI person—someone who
really enjoys working undercover!

FILE CLERK

ROASTS   He's so bad at his job, the only thing he should be
filing for is bankruptcy!

She's so bad at her work, she can't even file her own nails properly!

He had to go to a psychiatrist because he found himself eating alphabet soup in letter order!

Her husband is also seriously thinking of getting into filing—for divorce!

BOAST   I'm guaranteed to keep my job for a long time—I'm the only one in the office who knows the filing system!

TOAST   Here's a toast to a fine filing clerk—someone who has a terrific plan for losing things systematically!

FINANCIER

ROASTS   She really doesn't mind losing a lot of money in major investments as long as it isn't *her* money!

As a financier, he's the only man who can buy experience without actually paying for it himself!

She's obviously a determined financier, because she's always ready to back *her* decisions with *your* last cent!

He's obviously a financier—his wife never finds out when he gets a raise in salary!

BOAST   I know I'm a successful financier, because I always have my golf score above par and my stocks below it!

TOAST   Let's lift a toast to a financier who knows money doesn't talk nowadays—it goes without saying!

FIRE-EATER

ROASTS   Naturally, he's a fire-eater—you've never tasted his wife's cooking!

Obviously, she's a fire-eater, because she's always making an *ash* of herself!

Of course, he's a fire-eater because he makes light of everything!

The only way she'll ever get kissed will be if she gets asbestos lips!

BOAST   I never eat dynamite because I don't want to shoot my mouth off!

TOAST   Let's lift a toast to a terrific fire-eater, in fact, he's always matchless!

FIRE PERSON

ROASTS   Naturally, he's a fireman—people keep telling him to go to blazes!

She's so dumb, she thinks a fire engine is an engine that makes fires!

His wife is suing him for divorce because he's spending too much time with old flames!

She's so dumb, she wants to become Fire Commissioner so she can get a commission on each fire!

BOAST   I have a great idea for saving the department a lot of money—put unbreakable glass in all the fire alarms!

TOAST   Here's a toast to a fine fireman—someone who's always looking for a hot time!

FISHING PERSON

ROASTS   You can easily tell she's a fishing person, because she's such a *reel* sport!

You can easily tell he's a fisherman, because he always knows where to draw the line!

She started her profession early by fishing through ice—but all she got were olives and cherries!

He came by his profession naturally, because he's always been up to something fishy!

BOAST   I enjoy my job so much, during my time off I always go fishing!

TOAST   Let's lift a toast to a great fishing person—someone who always works for scale!

FLIGHT ATTENDANT

ROASTS   She knows how to handle rowdy children on her flights—she tells them to go outside and play!

He's always on an evening schedule—he works for a fly-by-night airline!

She's got a natural personality to be a stewardess—flighty!

He had to give up being a flight attendant—he's afraid of watching movies!

BOAST   I know I'm a terrific flight attendant—not one passenger has ever walked out on my service!

TOAST   Here's a toast to a dedicated flight attendant—he always seems to be up in the air about something!

FLORIST

ROASTS   He's a very secretive florist, quite *mum* about his work!

She's a high-pressure sales person—always trying to *petal* her posies!

He likes his women the same way he prefers his flowers—long-stemmed!

She's just like her flowers—she grows wild in the woods!

BOAST   I was an early success as a florist, but everyone knows it's a *budding* business!

TOAST   Here's a toast to a sex-crazed florist—just like his flowers, he's always found in beds!

FOREMAN

ROASTS   He may call himself a *fore*man, but *one* little old lady could do his job!

She's not only a foreman at work, she's also one nagging broad off the job!

If he thinks he's a good foreman, the jury will be out a heck of a long time on that one!

You can easily tell he's a foreman—that's how many men it takes to help him screw in a lightbulb!

BOAST   There's only one reason they call me a foreman—that's how many good men it would take to replace me!

TOAST   Let's lift a toast to a typical foreman—it only takes *four* drinks for him to pass out!

FORESTER

ROASTS   You can easily tell she's a forester because she's always going out on a limb!

You can easily tell he's forester because he's such a sap!

You can easily tell she's a forester because she's always barking up the wrong tree!

Even when he was a little boy, his father used to take him for long walks in the woods—and leave him there!

BOAST   I came up with a good idea for preventing forest fires— stomp out all the bears!

TOAST   Here's a toast to someone who knows how to prevent forest fires—he never lets cigarettes go out alone!

FORTUNE TELLER

ROASTS   You can easily tell he's a fortune teller—he likes to have everything done medium!

She may call herself a medium, but nothing she ever does is well-done!

He couldn't even translate the message in a Chinese fortune cookie!

The only spirits she's good at contacting come bottled!

BOAST   Not only is my face my good fortune, but I've also run it into a handsome figure!

TOAST   Let's lift a toast to a fine fortune teller—if anyone knows how to make an easy fortune, tell'er!

FRUIT PICKER

ROASTS   You can easily tell he's a fruit picker—he's *plum* crazy about his job!

She may be a good fruit picker, but when her husband chose her, he really picked a lemon!

He's so terrible at his job, he can't even pick his teeth properly!

You can easily tell she's a fruit picker—because she's always going out on a limb!

BOAST   I'm really dedicated to my job—I only wear Fruit-of-the-Looms!

TOAST   Here's a toast to a someone who really knows a lot about his work—he should, he's a real fruit!

FURNITURE MAKER

ROASTS   You can easily tell he's a furniture maker because he's always *board* with his work!

Her furniture making is realtively unknown because she works in the sticks!

He's terrible working on committees because he always wants to *table* everything!

She makes pretty good furniture, but her work needs a lot of polish!

BOAST   I make period furniture—the best that there is, that's all, *period*!

TOAST   Let's lift a toast to a fine furniture maker—someone who builds things we all bump in the night!

FURRIER

ROASTS   She always wears a lovely fur coat—she killed it herself!

He's so generous, he bought his wife a complete fur outfit—a steel trap and a rifle!

She knows what stands behind every successful man—a woman who wants a fur coat!

He just came up with a terrific idea for the everyday housewife—a wash-and-wear mink!

BOAST   I once sold to a customer who was so rich, she wanted a mink lining for her sable coat!

TOAST   Here's a toast to a someone who knows the true meaning of a fur coat— something given to a woman to keep her warm, or quiet!

G

GAMBLING DEALER

ROASTS   The reason he's such a terrible dealer is because he's not playing with a full deck!

The only sure bet in town right now is that she won't be able to keep her job!

He likes being a gambling dealer, otherwise he'd have to go out and work!

She looks just like she works her cards—badly stacked!

BOAST   I look and feel the age that's the same name as my favorite gambling game—twenty-one!

TOAST   Let's lift a toast to a gambling dealer whose life should be like her job—in the chips!

GARBAGE COLLECTOR

ROASTS   He actually enjoys being a garbage collector. If his cold ever clears up, he might change his mind!

At home, she doesn't use a garbage disposal—her husband takes care of that!

He likes to wake people up at five A.M. by making a lot of noise and then forget to take their garbage!

She constantly complains of being depressed because she's always down in the dumps!

BOAST   I enjoy my job so much, my idea of a big evening is to take out the garbage!

TOAST   Let's lift a toast to a true garbage collector—someone who always throws his trash out the window!

GARDENER

ROASTS   He may call himself a gardener but his wife calls him a blooming idiot!

She has a green thumb. That doesn't mean she's good at gardening— she really has a green thumb!

There's only one thing he manages to grow in his garden—tired!

She must be an excellent gardener. I heard she's still sowing her wild oats!

BOAST   I'm a gardener who really enjoys his work—I always dig what I'm doing!

TOAST   Let's lift a toast to a naturally good gardener—he's always potted!

GAS COMPANY PERSON

ROASTS   It's very easy to tell where she works—she's always emitting gas!

He obviously works for the gas company—he always acts like his pilot light isn't lit!

She's so dedicated to her job, she came to a Halloween party wearing a gas mask!

He's so dedicated to his job, even his television set is run by gas!

BOAST   A lot of people are envious of my job; exactly how many I don't know—I'd only be gassing!

TOAST   Here's a toast to someone who really enjoys his job—in fact, he thinks it's a real gas!

GENEALOGIST

ROASTS   He looked up his own family tree once and he found out he was only a sap!

She thought there might be some nobility in her own genealogical background, but she found she was barking up the wrong tree!

He specializes in tracing back your family—just as far as your money will go!

She's a true genealogist. In tracing your ancestry, she always finds people who were better than you are!

BOAST   I'm as good at genealogy as I am at gardening—I'm always watching my roots!

TOAST   Let's lift a toast to someone who is obviously a fine genealogist—always looking for alternate roots!

GEOLOGIST

ROASTS   He became a geologist quite naturally since he's always finding faults!

She told her dentist to go ahead and drill anyway, because she felt lucky!

You can tell he's a geologist—even his hair and skin are oily!

I don't know why she has so much trouble finding oil. You can buy it at the filling station for less than a dollar a can!

BOAST   I became a geologist quite naturally because I'm such a down-to-earth fellow!

TOAST   Here's a toast to a true geologist—she yearns the midday oil!

GLASS BLOWER

ROASTS   She's true to her profession—she blows every job she gets!

He got fired from his last job—he had a bad case of hiccups and blew nothing but crystal balls!

She has a lot of trouble keeping jobs—she likes to whistle while she works!

He's so terrible in his job, he couldn't even blow his nose properly!

BOAST   When I retire from my job, I'm going to have a really big blow-out!

TOAST   Here's a toast to a person who is truly dedicated to his job—he always blows his paycheck!

GLASS INSTALLER

ROASTS   He was fired from his last job. . . after a really shattering experience!

She's a very particular glass installer—she doesn't do windows!

His wife knows he works with glass—she can always see right through him!

She reminds you of the glass she installs—a real pane!

BOAST   After a hard day's work, the only glass I'm interested in holds a pitcher of beer!

TOAST   Let's lift a toast to an installer who only does quality work—someone with a real *glass* act!

GOVERNMENT WORKER

ROASTS   Her job with the government has influenced her new hobby—working on a perpetual motion machine!

He has a hobby that was influenced by working in the government—grafting!

She should be very good working for the government—she's always involved in a state of affairs!

He works for a government bureau—that's where the taxpayers' shirts are kept!

BOAST   I like working for the government—it employs some of the best people money can buy!

TOAST   Here's a toast to a fine goverment worker—someone who works for a system that regards a citizen as one who has what it takes!

GRAPHOLOGIST

ROASTS   He knew he was destined to be a graphologist when he saw the handwriting on the wall!

Her own handwriting is so terrible, the only way she can get a message across is to type it!

You can easily tell he's a handwriting expert—because he's always well-looped!

She may be an expert on handwriting, but she still has to learn one thing—how to read!

BOAST   I can do something that a lot of other people can't—read my own handwriting!

TOAST   Let's lift a toast to a fine handwriting expert—someone to whom life is one long sentence!

GRINDER

ROASTS   Her very first job as a grinder ended rather abruptly—her monkey died!

His wife says that living with him every day is the real grind!

Take one good look at her face and you can tell she keeps her nose to the grindstone!

His real grind is getting himself to the shop after a heavy night on the town!

BOAST   I'm so involved with my job, when I sleep I grind my teeth!

TOAST   Here's a toast to a true grinder—always worrying about his organ!

GROCER

ROASTS   You can easily tell he's a grocer—he's always in the market for something!

You can easily tell she's a grocer—she's always carting around!

I bought fifty dollars worth of food at his market, and somebody stole it out of my glove compartment!

The food prices are so deadly at her market she gives *black* stamps!

BOAST   I don't know about the rest of you folks, but I'm doing just great in the market!

TOAST   Let's lift a toast to a great grocer who runs a fine market—a place you can go broke shopping in just one store!

GROOM

ROASTS   With her looks, she might as well call herself a groom—she'll never be a *bride*!

You can easily tell he's a groom by the way he likes to horse around!

People say that she reminds them of clouds because she likes to hold the reins!

He's great at grooming horses. Now he should do something about grooming himself!

BOAST   I may be a confirmed bachelor, but I'll always be a groom!

TOAST   Here's a toast to a great groom—someone who has a lot of horsepower!

GUARD

ROASTS   He's so terrible at his job, he couldn't guard against body odor!

There's only one security she should worry about—keeping her job!

Whenever his wife gets mad at him, she puts him in the guardhouse!

To show you how good she is, her last job was guarding Jimmy Hoffa!

BOAST   The reason I'm so great at my job is because every morning before going to work I use Right Guard!

TOAST   Let's lift a toast to a terrific guard—someone who never lets his job interfere with catching up on his sleep!

H

HAIRDRESSER

ROASTS   A woman once spent three hours in her chair—and that was just for the estimate!

When he sets hair, people in the shop wonder when it will go off!

She believes in the beautician's motto: hair today, gone tomorrow!

He made one girl look like a real doll—her hair was pasted on!

BOAST   I can make your hair so curly, people will get seasick just looking at it!

TOAST   Here's a toast to a dedicated hairdresser—every day, she just dyes to get to work!

HEALTH WORKER

ROASTS   She obviously got into her job for the money—certainly *not* for her health!

His own wife's health has him worried—it's always good!

She may be a good health worker, but her face makes you sick!

He's seriously thinking of quitting his job—he's *bored* of health!

BOAST   I may quit my health job because of illness and fatigue—I'm sick and tired of it!

TOAST   Here's a toast to someone who always does her job well—if she knows what's good for her health!

HERPETOLOGIST

ROASTS   You can easily tell he's a herpetologist because he works for scale!

You can easily tell she's a herpetologist—she doesn't walk to work, she slithers!

His wife knew just what to buy him for Christmas—a pair of slithers!

You can easily tell he's a herpetologist—he's always trying to make the bite on you!

BOAST   I get along great with the reptiles I study—they all look up to me!

TOAST   Let's lift a toast to a great herpetologist—someone who always has a good grip on his work!

HISTORIAN

ROASTS   Study for her was easy in the beginning—at that time, there was *no* history!

If you want to hear some real surprises of history, he should reveal his own!

Studying history for her was easy—she's lived through all of it!

He may know a lot about history, but there's no future to his job!

BOAST   I think the history of the world proves we should be coming to peace instead of going to pieces!

TOAST   Here's a toast to a true historian, just like his subject, he's always repeating himself!

HOG CALLER

ROASTS   He's so fat, he should call himself!

She even does her job while driving her car—she's a road hog caller!

He started calling hogs for only one reason—he was desperate for a date!

If you don't like the way she calls hogs, you should hear the way she calls her husband!

BOAST   I'm so crazy about my hog calling job, I just wallow in it!

TOAST   Let's lift a toast to a really great hog caller—he's so good at his job, they have to keep him penned!

HOOKER

ROASTS   She's been picked up so many times, she's beginning to grow handles!

She was fired by her pimp for *not* laying down on the job!

Her mother knows she's a hooker, but she always tells friends that her daughter makes rugs!

She may be a loose woman, but she always finds herself in a tight squeeze!

BOAST   I'm a girl who doesn't give all to love, because I give love to all—for a price!

TOAST   Let's lift a toast to a true hooker—she knows more sailors than an admiral!

HOSPITAL WORKER

ROASTS   You can easily tell she's a hospital worker by her bed-pan expression!

As a hospital worker, he has few friends and a lot of enemas!

She decided to get a job at the hospital, so she could visit her bills!

He belongs in a hospital—he's a real sickie!

BOAST   I like working in a hospital—it's the place people who are run down usually wind up!

TOAST   Here's a toast to a real hospital worker—someone who must have a lot of patients!

HOTEL MANAGER

ROASTS   The one thing he manages best is to keep the hotel owners fooled about what he's really doing!

She manages to spend more time drinking in the bar than any of the guests!

He managed a hotel where business was so bad, the owners stole towels from the guests!

Her guests never complain about the room service—there's never any to complain about!

BOAST   I once managed a hotel that was so ritzy, we wouldn't let anyone into the steamroom without a tie and jacket!

TOAST   Let's lift a toast to a manager who's worked a lot of different hotels—he's got the towels and silverware to prove it!

HOUSE PAINTER

ROASTS   She's so terrible a painter, she even has to paint houses by the number!

He's so terrible at his job, the only houses he's fit to paint are *out*-houses!

She's so terrible at her job, she could mess up the color on the White House!

He started painting houses after his wife gave him the brush!

BOAST   I'm so crazy about my job, for my vacation I went to the Painted Desert!

TOAST   Here's a toast to a very thorough house painter—he even paints the windows—not the sills, the actual windows!

HOUSEKEEPER

ROASTS   When it comes to good housekeeping, he likes to do nothing better!

She has something that does all the housework for her—a husband!

The owner of the house is lucky the housekeeper is terrible at fixing things. . . everything works!

She once kept a house that was so far in the sticks, the mailman sent the mail there by mail!

BOAST   I know I'm a great housekeeper—everytime I get a divorce, I keep the house!

TOAST   Let's lift a toast to a housekeeper who doesn't know the meaning of the word dust—because she never sees any!

HYPNOTIST

ROASTS   She hypnotized her husband into thinking he was a chicken—because they needed the eggs!

His hypnosis business was so bad, *he* was the only one who went under!

She never finished her hypnosis lessons in school—during class she fell asleep!

He asked a patient under hypnosis to act like a Princess and she rang like a telephone!

BOAST   I'm such a great hypnotist, I convinced my wife to stop using her credit cards!

TOAST   Here's a toast to a terrific hypnotist—someone who discovered a great cure for amnesia, but he forgot what it was!

I

ICHTHYOLOGIST

ROASTS   I suspected he was an ichthylogist because there's always been something fishy about him!

She's such a terrible ichthyologist, she can't even open a can of sardines!

He's so crazy about ichthyology that his favorite hobby is fishing!

She thinks she's such a great ichthyologist—she's always fishing for compliments!

BOAST   I don't make a lot of money as an ichthyologist. I only work for scale!

TOAST   Let's lift a toast to a well-educated ichthyologist—someone who's gone to a lot of schools!

IMPORTER

ROASTS   The only thing he should import is a new set of brains for himself!

The reason she's such a great importer is because she has so many foreign affairs!

He's so dumb, he's importing ice cubes from Alaska for mixed drinks!

She's cornered the market on a great new item she's importing— wash-and-wear mink!

BOAST   I'm now importing period furniture—I keep it for a period, then send it back!

TOAST   Here's a toast to an importer who likes dealing with red China. Too bad it doesn't match the tablecloth!

INDIAN CHIEF

ROASTS   He just got a new job with the sign department in the city Traffic Bureau—designing arrows!

You can easily tell he's an Indian Chief—he's wearing an Arrow shirt!

There's been some doubt expressed about his leadership ability— many of his people have their reservations!

He may be the Indian Chief, but it's his wife who always seems to be on the warpath!

BOAST   I once decided to set my feather warbonnet on fire—to keep my *wig-wam!*

TOAST   Let's lift a toast to a very smart Indian Chief—only he knows what he *really* smokes in that peace pipe!

INSPECTOR

ROASTS   As a teenager, whenever she came home late from a date, her mother would "inspect'er!"

He learned all his bungling on the job by watching old Pink Panther movies!

The one big thing she should really inspect is obvious—herself!

If anybody ever bothered to inspect his brain, they'd find it empty!

BOAST   As for myself, I never need inspection—because I don't have any defects!

TOAST   Here's a toast to a fine inspector—someone whose prime interest is inspecting his pay envelope!

INSURANCE PERSON

ROASTS   The only insurance he really can't get is that he'll keep his job!

She offers a special policy if you accidentally get hit on the head—they pay you a lump sum!

He doesn't carry life insurance; he has fire insurance instead. He knows where he's going!

She offers an exclusive new fire and theft insurance. You only get paid if your house is robbed while it's burning!

BOAST   I now have a brand new double indemity policy. If you die in an accident, we bury you twice!

TOAST   Here's a toast to the insurance man's motto: the big print giveth, and the small print taketh away!

INTERIOR DECORATOR

ROASTS   She's so dumb, she swallowed a gallon of paint so she could decorate her interior!

He always crowds a home with atmosphere and the owners give him the air!

She should do all her rooms in stripes, because the way she decorates is a crime!

He claims all his furniture goes back to Henry the Eighth—next week it goes back to Sears!

BOAST   I'm a very meticulous interior decorator—I even put drapes on the TV screen!

TOAST   Here's a toast to a very expensive interior decorator—someone who always thinks you inherited your money!

INTERPRETER

ROASTS   He has such a heavy foreign accent, you need an interpreter to interpret the interpreter!

She's such a great interpreter because she's had so many international relations!

He has a perfect system for interpreting words he really doesn't understand—he mumbles!

She wears such terrible-looking clothes, she needs to learn the interpretation of good taste!

BOAST   I'm such a great interpreter, I even understand everything my wife has to say!

TOAST   Let's lift a toast to a great interpreter—he even understands all the deductions on his paycheck!

INVENTOR

ROASTS   She crossed a mink with a gorilla to breed ready-made fur coats but the sleeves were too long!

He invented a mattress with an automatic toaster built in it so you can pop out of bed in the morning!

She invented pancakes that contain popcorn so they can flip over by themselves!

He invented cigarettes with dynamite in them for people who like to shoot their mouths off!

BOAST   I just invented a television set with a screen seventeen inches wide and two inches high. It's for people who squint!

TOAST   Here's a toast to a typical inventor—someone who works long and hard on gadgets that will save work!

INVENTORY WORKER

ROASTS   He's so dumb, somebody should take inventory of his head—for brains!

She's so involved with her work, everytime she goes to the supermarket, she starts taking inventory!

If the company ever took inventory of how much work he does, he'd be fired!

If the company really wants an accurate account of their inventory, they should check her house!

BOAST   If anybody ever tried to list my wonderful assets they'd find an endless inventory!

TOAST   Let's lift a toast to a terrific inventory worker—someone in whom we can take a lot of stock!

J

JAILER

ROASTS   You can easily tell she's a jailer because she spends so much time in front of bars!

He should really be a writer because he's in charge of so many sentences!

She's so dumb, she keeps a parakeet in the cells as a jailbird!

He's becoming quite government educated talking with all the jailed politicians!

BOAST   I know I'm a successful jailer because my prisoners are always keyed up!

TOAST   Here's a toast to a truly sentimental jailer—someone who always hates to see you go!

JANITOR

ROASTS   Naturally, he's a janitor—as a hobby he collects dust!

Obviously, she's a janitor because she acts crazy with the heat!

You can easily tell he's the janitor because he'd rather sleep than heat!

Naturally, she's the janitor because she's known by the temperature she keeps!

BOAST   Most people think janitors don't make much money, but I'm really cleaning up!

TOAST   Let's lift a toast to a typical janitor—the last person to know there's been a drop in the temperature!

JEWELER

ROASTS   His wife dropped the diamond ring he gave her and she had seven years bad luck!

She's so dumb a jeweler, she doesn't know any facet of her job!

With the divorce rate nowadays, he's starting to *rent* wedding rings!

The only diamond she knows anything about is at the baseball stadium!

BOAST   I know I'm a great jeweler because everyone says I'm a real gem!

TOAST   Let's lift a toast to a jeweler who really knows his stones—if he knew anything about jewelry he'd be great!

JOCKEY

ROASTS   You can easily tell she's a jockey because she's always running around in circles!

He's so terrible a jockey, on weekends he hires himself out to pose on people's front lawns!

She once rode a horse that took so long to come in, instead of using a stopwatch they used a calendar!

He once rode a horse that was so far behind, they had to photograph the track again several times to find him!

BOAST   I know that I'm a jockey—to prove it, all you have to do is read the label in my shorts!

TOAST   Here's a toast to a dedicated jockey—on his day off, he goes horseback riding!

JUDGE

ROASTS   She once handed down a judgement that was so complex, nobody knew what the judge *meant*!

He handed down so many decisions, he became a case-hardened individual!

You can easily tell she's a judge because she's always in a trying position!

You can easily tell he's a judge because he's a man of many convictions!

BOAST   I like handing out sentences, because I figure it's more blessed to give than to receive!

TOAST   Let's lift a toast to a typical judge—it's really his wife who lays down the law!

K

KENNEL KEEPER

ROASTS   Some folks once asked her to keep a kangaroo, but they left her holding the bag!

His business is so bad, the kennel is really going to the dogs!

You can easily tell she likes to take care of dogs because she goes for anything in pants!

There are so many dogs boarded at the kennel, his business is really picking up!

BOAST   I worked so hard at the kennel today, I came home dog tired!

TOAST   Here's a toast to a kennel keeper who learned a lot about dogs from his wife—she taught him how to beg!

L

LAB TECHNICIAN

ROASTS   She had nothing to do in the lab the other day—she lost her test tube scrubber!

He's a typical lab technician—always putting off until tomorrow what he can put off for good!

She may think she's a great technician at the lab, but her outside life couldn't take being examined under a microscope!

He got fired from his last job for thinking too big. . . at a transistor firm!

BOAST   I'm really dedicated to my job. At home, I show friends my microscopic slides!

TOAST   Let's lift a toast to a great lab technician. It's just too bad he can't brew a decent cup of coffee!

LAND DEVELOPER

ROASTS   He's a terrific land developer. Now if only he could develop some business ethics to go along with it!

Some developer she is—she couldn't develop a roll of film if she took it to the drugstore!

He's just great at developing land—where the land usually develops termites!

She has good reason for being distracted lately—she has a *lot* on her mind!

BOAST   I'm a very grateful land developer—I truly have *lots* to be thankful for!

TOAST   Here's a toast to someone who's always interested in land—landing a good deal, that is!

LATHE OPERATOR

ROASTS   He's obviously a lathe operator—that's why his head is always in a spin!

She met her husband while he was also operating a lathe and they've been going around together ever since!

He's obviously a lathe operator because he's always giving cutting remarks!

She's obviously a lathe operator by the way she keeps rotating from one job to another!

BOAST   I'm really dedicated to my job. Even after work, I like tooling around!

TOAST   Let's lift a toast to a fine lathe operator—someone who always likes making the rounds!

LAUNDRY WORKER

ROASTS   She's such a neurotic laundry worker, she keeps losing her buttons!

He's such a terrible laundry worker, the customers call him Jack the Ripper!

She's obviously a terrible laundry worker—everything she does is off the cuff!

He just got a notice from the Board of Health. . . to clean up his act!

BOAST   I have a lot of friends in my business—they literally give me the shirts off their backs!

TOAST   Here's a toast to a laundry worker with many rivals—someone who always has clothes competition!

LEATHER WORKER

ROASTS   Obviously, he's a leather worker. Instead of pajamas for bed, he wears chaps!

She came by her job quite naturally, even her skin looks and feels like leather!

He's obviously a leather worker—instead of chairs in his home, he has saddles!

She came by her job quite naturally—even in her conversation, she's always stretching things!

BOAST   Obviously, I'm a great leather worker—I always have such a great tan!

TOAST   Let's lift a toast to a mean leather worker—someone who's always taking things out on your hide!

LECTURER

ROASTS   She may be a terrible lecturer on the podium, but she's terrific with her husband at home!

He speaks straight from the shoulder, but he'd be a lot more interesting if his thoughts came from a little higher up!

She'd be a great lecturer about the topic she knows best—hot air!

As a lecturer, his vocabulary is small but the turnover is terrific!

BOAST   I'm such a great lecturer, everyone calls me "Amazon" because I'm so big at the mouth!

TOAST   Here's a toast to a great lecturer of a few words—a few million of them!

LEGAL SECRETARY

ROASTS   He's a legal secretary—that means he didn't have enough money to go to law school!

She must be having an affair with her boss. She's always talking about helping him with his briefs!

He's obviously a legal secretary—his favorite card game is contract bridge!

She's obviously a legal secretary, because she has to work with a lot of will!

BOAST   I'm a truly great legal secretary because I always tailor a terrific lawsuit!

TOAST   Let's lift a toast to a great legal secretary—someone who's main job is typing out her boss's words and anger!

LIBRARIAN

ROASTS   As a librarian, silence isn't just golden to her—it's a living!

You can easily tell he's a librarian—with him, good looks are long overdue!

She's obviously a librarian—you can read her like a book!

He's stolen so many books from work, whenever you enter his house you have to show your library card!

BOAST   There's only one thing that frustrates me about my library job—I can't whistle while I work!

TOAST   Here's a toast to a great librarian—someone who does a superb job at keeping the books!

LIFEGUARD

ROASTS   He saved several lives at the beach yesterday—he didn't show up for work!

She started out her job quite slowly—as a lifeguard at a carwash!

He really likes the beach. It's a place where people lie on the sand—about how well they're doing in life!

She likes to walk along the beach, slap people on the back and ask them how they're peeling!

BOAST   I'm so good looking when I walk onto the beach, even the tide refuses to go out!

TOAST   Let's lift a toast to a fine lifeguard. The only lifesaver she knows anything about comes in five flavors!

LIGHTING TECHNICIAN

ROASTS   He's obviously a lighting technician because he likes to put the shine on people!

She may think she's a great lighting technician, but her future is looking dim!

He had so much to drink the other night, he went out like one of his lights!

She may think she's a great lighting technician, but in the brain department she's not very bright!

BOAST   There's a basic reason why I'm so terrific at my job—it's because I'm so light-hearted!

TOAST   Let's lift a toast to a lighting technician who knows his job because he follows all the current events!

LINEMAN

ROASTS   I wouldn't want to say she's an overweight lineman, but lately she keeps climbing the poles into the ground!

It's obvious what he does for a living, because he's so good at handing people a line!

She's obviously a lineman, because she always seems to be up to something!

He might seem to write good work reports, but you have to read between his lines!

BOAST   I know I'm great at my job—because people keep whistling at my lines!

TOAST   Here's a toast to a fine lineman—someone whose greatest lines are in his face!

LINGUIST

ROASTS   If you think he knows linguistics, you should hear some of the language he uses around his house!

Some of the language she uses is so bad, she should go back to grammar school!

He's such a terrible linguist everything he says is tongue-in-cheek!

She only studied linguistics for one reason—so she could tell dialect jokes!

BOAST   As a true linguist, I may not always know what a word means, but I always know how to pronounce it!

TOAST   Let's lift a toast to a true linguist—someone who always has the time to argue a word with you!

LION TAMER

ROASTS   She's so terrible at her work, the lion sits in the chair and whips *her*!

I tried to call him at work the other day, but the *lion* was busy!

She's such a terrible lion tamer—she always looks down in the mouth!

He was such a brat as a child, everybody said he'd end up behind bars!

BOAST   I was destined to be a lion tamer from birth. My mother was at an M-G-M movie at the time!

TOAST   Here's a toast to a real cool lion tamer—someone who always hangs around with a lot of cats!

LIQUOR PERSON

ROASTS   Naturally, he's in the liquor business—he's a certified alcoholic!

Her customers don't mind being charged a liquor tax—they're all too drunk to care!

I wouldn't want to say his liquor is cheap, but it's just great for rubdowns!

She sells a new whisky toothpaste. You get 25 percent more cavities, but you don't give a damn!

BOAST   I just started a new customer pickup service—to drive people to drink!

TOAST   Let's lift a toast to a great liquor person—someone who's always with fine spirits!

LOAN OFFICER

ROASTS   Whenever a caller asks for the Lone Arranger, she always expects them to say, "Let-a me speak-a to Tonto!"

I wouldn't want to say he's a loan shark, but his customers call him "Jaws!"

She only works for the principle of the thing, and takes a lot of interest in doing it!

He's so stingy, he won't even loan out a book without a first trust deed!

BOAST   I just thought of a new home loan market. . . for customers at the supermarket checkout!

TOAST   Here's a toast to a great loan officer—I wouldn't even let him borrow my lawn mower!

LOCKSMITH

ROASTS   He's so terrible at his job, the only thing he could pick is his teeth!

She comes by her locksmith job quite naturally, because she's always so keyed up!

His breath is so bad, the best thing for him would be lock*jaw*!

She's a Jewish locksmith—whenever she goes to a deli, she orders lox!

BOAST   I'm such a great locksmith even when I sing, I'm right on key!

TOAST   Let's lift a toast to a great locksmith—someone who's made a fortune with a coat hanger and an ice pick!

LOGGER

ROASTS   She used to call trees her friends until she fell out of one of her friends!

He's not mean enough to bite you, but you'd better watch out for his bark!

She complains about her job as a logger, because business has been falling off lately!

He's so dumb a logger he'll climb out on a limb to saw it off!

BOAST   I'm doing so well in the logging business, I'm thinking of opening a branch office!

TOAST   Here's a toast to a great logger—someone who's made a fortune just lumbering along!

LUGGAGE HANDLER

ROASTS   He's so terrible at his job, he doesn't just handle your luggage—he *mangles* it!

She always knows where your luggage is if you ask her—it's lost!

You can tell he's a luggage handler from the bags under his eyes!

They just gave her a very appropriate job: handling old bags!

BOAST   I'm so great at my job that last week I finally found Amelia Earhart's luggage!

TOAST   Let's lift a toast to a true luggage handler—someone to whom everything is an open and unshut case!

M

MACHINIST

ROASTS   He has a terrible reputation as a machinist—always grabbing other people's tools!

She's always complaining about her job because it's such a grind!

His personality is just like his machinist job—always boring!

She may be a lady machinist, but she's used to a lot of shavings!

BOAST   I enjoy my job so much as a machinist, even after work I like milling around!

TOAST   Let's lift a toast to a true machinist—someone who is always making cutting remarks!

MAGICIAN

ROASTS   She's a natural magician—people keep asking her to disappear!

Naturally, she's a magician, because she's a very difficult person to conjure with.

He thinks he's such a great magician, but the only thing he can't make disappear are his bills!

She's obviously a magician because she's always got something up her sleeve!

BOAST   I've just thought up a terrific new magic trick—pulling a hat out of a rabbit!

TOAST   Here's a toast to a great magician—he performs tricks even a kid will believe!

MAID

ROASTS   She's such a terrible maid, she cleans everyone out of house and home!

She's such a mean maid, she short-sheets every bed in the house!

She's such a careless maid, she's what you'd call worse for the dinnerware!

She's a maid who can't keep a secret, but she's used to spilling the beans!

BOAST   I'm such a dedicated maid, I only drink wine that's domestic!

TOAST   Let's lift a toast to a great maid—the only way to get a glass of water from her is to set yourself on fire!

MAILROOM WORKER

ROASTS   It's obvious when she works in the company, because she's only interested in the *males*!

He's such a terrible mailroom worker, he might find out that it's not just the letters that are subject to cancellation!

Her favorite pastime in the mailroom is holding up company pay envelopes to the light!

He complains all day about pigeon-holing letters, because he wants a job of a different sort!

BOAST   I'm a person of many letters. . . even though they belong to the company!

TOAST   Here's a toast to a dedicated mailroom worker—someone who either likes his job or collecting stamps!

MANICURIST

ROASTS   She's a manicurist who was once married to a dentist, but they fought tooth and nail!

She has her own special method of doing her own nails—she bites them!

She believes in a manicurist marriage—when it's time for divorce, she files!

She charges so much for a manicure, her customers really get clipped!

BOAST   I'm such a successful manicurist, I make money hand over fist!

TOAST   Let's lift a toast to a really successful manicurist—she makes money every time she lifts a finger!

MANUFACTURER

ROASTS   I have no idea what he makes in his factory, but it certainly isn't money!

The only thing she's good at manufacturing are excuses for doing such terrible business!

He's great at manufacturing—when it comes time to explain to his wife why he came home so late!

She went broke manufacturing bowling balls without holes in them— for people who don't like to bowl!

BOAST   I make a fortune manufacturing books with blank pages in them—for people who don't like to read!

TOAST   Here's a toast to a failure as a snuff manufacturer— someone who was always putting his business in other people's noses!

MARINE

ROASTS   He used to be an oil rig operator before he joined the Marines. . . so they made him a drill sargeant!

They told him that he wasn't good enough to be a Marine. . . so they made him a *sub*-Marine!

He's so terrible a Marine, he shouldn't be in a landing force, he belongs in a landing *farce*!

He's such a dedicated Marine, he even likes eating creamed chipped beef on toast!

BOAST   I'm such a dedicated Marine, my favorite month of the year is a long March!

TOAST   Let's lift a toast to a man who fought with the Marines— he couldn't get along with anybody!

MARKETING SPECIALIST

ROASTS   Some Marketing Specialist! She got all her training at the A & P!

The only marketing he knows anything about comes on a grocery list!

Her first advice as a Marketing Specialist is to save Green Stamps!

He knows all about marketing—his wife showed him how at the neighborhood Safeway!

BOAST   I have a new idea to market large, edible pillows—for people who like to dream of giant marshmallows at night!

TOAST   Here's a toast to the first man to market radio dinners—for people who don't own TV sets!

MARRIAGE COUNSELOR

ROASTS   He isn't just an expensive marriage counselor—he's constantly torn between love and booty!

She naturally became a marriage counselor—she used to be a referee!

He's such a terrible marriage counselor that he and his wife schedule a regular fight-of-the-week!

She knows that the most foolish woman can manage a clever man, but it takes a very clever woman to manage a fool!

BOAST   My simple advice to husbands: it's always safer to tease a dog than a woman!

TOAST   Let's lift a toast to a true marriage counselor—someone who specializes in untying slip knots!

MASSAGER

ROASTS   She keeps getting fired from her job as a massager—for rubbing people the wrong way!

He quite naturally became a massager, because he's always rubbing it in!

She's always complaining about her job as a massager—working her fingers to other people's bones!

He quite naturally became a massager—he's very good at manipulating people!

BOAST   I know I'm a great massager because I'm an expert at *fats* and figures!

TOAST   Here's a toast to a great massager—someone who always recognizes a knead!

MATHEMATICIAN

ROASTS   He's such a terrible mathematician—his whole life adds up to a complete mess!

She's obviously a mathematician—she only likes to plant square roots!

He's such a terrible mathematician that he can't explain what happens to a man if his wife is his better half and he marries twice!

She's such a terrible mathematician that she'd give a thousand dollars to become a millionaire!

BOAST   I get such a thrill from mathematics—I just love to divide and conquer!

TOAST   Let's lift a toast to a true mathematician—someone who has the most trouble balancing his checkbook!

MECHANIC

ROASTS   She likes to tell people that if their car was a horse it would have to be shot!

He's a mechanic who can make your auto go fast—and your money go faster!

She has good advice if your hubcaps keep coming off: let some air out of your tires!

With his high repair bills, your car can keep you strapped without seatbelts!

BOAST   As an expert mechanic, I know the most dangerous part of an automobile—the nut behind the steering wheel!

TOAST   Here's a toast to a true mechanic—someone who advises customers to keep the oil and change the car!

MERCHANT

ROASTS   He specializes in selling things below cost that somehow he bought still further below cost!

She recently had a big fire sale—three big fires set for a hundred dollars!

He's having a special sale on old wind-up telephones—for people who make crank calls!

She may call herself a lady merchant, but people who shop in her store call her a counter-irritant!

BOAST   I'm thinking of opening a unique dimestore—some-place where you can actually buy something for under a dollar!

TOAST   Let's lift a toast to a fine merchant—someone who just needs a little wind taken out of his sales!

MESSENGER

ROASTS   She's often the messenger of bad news—something called good when worse happens!

He quit his job when he found out what ancient kings used to do with bearers of bad news—kill the messenger!

Her delivery is so slow, she even gets beat by the U.S. Post Office!

He's so terrible at his job, he'd have trouble delivering a message to himself!

BOAST   I was born to be a messenger—I came by special de-livery!

TOAST   Here's a toast to someone who's always in a hurry—especially to get out the door at quitting time!

METALLURGIST

ROASTS   He's an iron and steel man—his wife irons and he steals!

She came by her job quite naturally—she likes to *mettle* in other people's business!

Naturally, he's a metallurgist—he has lots of gold in his teeth and plenty of silver in his hair!

She just bought a huge crate of steel wool to knit herself a stove!

BOAST   I'm a dedicated metallurgist—you should see my collection of beer cans!

TOAST   Let's lift a toast to a true metallurgist—he knows how to say and spell the word "aluminum!"

MIDWIFE

ROASTS   She's so dumb, she thinks a midwife is a woman who's between husbands!

You can tell she's a midwife—even her conversation has a lot of pregnant pauses!

She's quite naturally a midwife—she always seems to be in hot water!

Keeping her job as a midwife requires mainly one thing—a lot of pull!

BOAST   Every day I work as a midwife it's the same holiday—Labor Day!

TOAST   Here's a toast to a fine midwife—someone who specializes in special deliveries!

MILK DELIVERER

ROASTS   He's such a lazy milkman, the amount of work he does is *udderly* ridiculous!

She's quite naturally a milk deliverer—she looks like a cow!

He had to quit his last job as a milkman—everything was going sour!

She's so dumb, the only kind of milk she knows anything about is milk of magnesia!

BOAST   The milk I deliver is so fresh, just three hours before it was grass!

TOAST   Let's lift a toast to a clever milk deliverer. To keep the milk from going sour, he keeps it in the cow!

MIME

ROASTS   She's quite naturally a mime—she's used to giving her husband the silent treatment!

He's so dumb a mime, he keeps trying to get his act on the radio!

Her mime act is so terrible, people prefer viewing it in the dark!

He once lost his job while performing his act—for shouting, "Fire!"

BOAST   I actually became a mime quite by accident—right before I came onstage, I got laryngitis!

TOAST   Here's a toast to a fine mime—someone whose own talent leaves him speechless!

MINER

ROASTS   He's so dumb, he thought the easiest job he could get would be mining *soft* coal!

She's so dumb, she thinks being a miner in this state makes her age under twenty-one!

He may be a miner, but he goes to great depths to give people a bad time!

She's obviously a miner—one good look and you can tell she's a gold-digger!

BOAST   There's only one reason I'm a miner—I really dig what I'm doing!

TOAST   Let's lift a toast to a fine miner—may he never be given the shaft!

MORTICIAN

ROASTS   His mortuary is so modern, they have hot and cold running formaldehyde!

She never has trouble working out payments for the deceased's family—she has a special layaway plan!

He has a very popular mortuary—people are just dying to get in there!

She closes all her letters with, "Eventually Yours!"

BOAST   I just ran a very popular radio commercial for my mortuary—60 seconds of dead air!

TOAST   Here's a toast to the mortician's motto: Life is wonderful; without it, you're dead!

MOVER

ROASTS   There's only one kind of moving she really enjoys—moving pictures!

If you want some easy firewood, just ask him to help you move your furniture!

She had to quit her last moving job because of illness—dropsy!

He had to quit his last position because of emotional stress—each job was a moving experience!

BOAST   I've had a lot of moving experience—I always skip out on my rent!

TOAST   Here's a toast to someone with the will to move mountains. Too bad he can't move furniture without breaking any!

MUSEUM WORKER

ROASTS   He's so old a museum worker, he should be one of the exhibits!

She decided to remove a painting in her museum—the artist had missed one of the numbers!

He thought his wife looked as pretty as a picture—so he hung her in his museum!

The lighting in her museum is so bad, the exhibit signs are written in Braille!

BOAST   My first job was working part-time at a Wax Museum—
only on *wick*-ends!

TOAST   Let's lift a toast to a fine museum worker—someone
whose best friend is his mummy!

MUSHROOM GROWER

ROASTS   She's a natural mushroom grower—always digging for
dirt!

He's a natural mushroom grower—his head has always been in the
dark!

She learned the difference between mushrooms and toadstools from
a dear friend—a dear, *departed* friend!

He has a special place in his house for love-making. He calls it his
mush room!

BOAST   I grow mushrooms so big, just one of them in my cellar
doesn't allow for *mush* room!

TOAST   Here's a toast to a true mushroom grower—without a
crop, he wouldn't know how to stew!

MUSICIAN

ROASTS   He's been having a lot of trouble with his guitar lately—
people keep hitting him over his head with it!

She puts her instrument in the refrigerator so she can play it cool!

He doesn't play piano by ear, he plays it by the window to annoy the neighbors!

She broke open her drum just to look inside and see what was making all the noise!

BOAST   Some say as a musician I'm finished. But I claim I'm a finished musician!

TOAST   Let's lift a toast to a true musician—he plays the "Minute Waltz" like there's no tomorrow!

N

NAVIGATOR

ROASTS   His real navigational challenge is getting home after a few beers!

She's so terrible at her job, she can't even navigate her car into a parking space!

He hasn't any sense at all, yet alone a sense of direction!

She's such a terrible navigator, she needs a compass to find the bathroom in her own house!

BOAST   There's one phrase I'm really sick and tired of hearing: "See you later, navigator!"

TOAST   Let's lift a toast to a true navigator—someone we should all steer clear of!

NAVY PERSON

ROASTS   She was once classified as a naval surgeon. My, some doctors really specialize, don't they?

He became so used to being in the Navy, off shore he slept on a waterbed!

She's so dumb, she thinks a naval destroyer is a hula-hoop with a nail in it!

He proposed to his wife while in the service—it was a naval engagement!

BOAST   While in the Navy, I was the only survivor when my ship got sunk. I missed the boat!

TOAST   Here's a toast to a true Navy person—someone who gets seasick taking a bath!

NEWS PERSON

ROASTS   He's so dumb, the only things that he knows are "current" are jams and jellies!

The only thing she thinks is big news is when she gets a raise!

The editor gave her the police beat, because the way she writes is such a crime!

Yesterday, he came in with two scoops—one vanilla and one strawberry!

BOAST   I used to be an old newspaper man, but I couldn't make any money selling old newspapers!

TOAST   Let's lift a toast to a fine news person—someone whose reporting covers a multitude of sins!

NIGHTCLUB OPERATOR

ROASTS   She's a terrible nightclub operator—she always gets smashed before the customers do!

His nightclub is such a dump, it looks like an ashtray with music!

The people in her club get so loaded, instead of a night spot it's a *tight* spot!

His nightclub is so rowdy, the tables are reserved but the customers aren't!

BOAST   At my nightclub we check people's hats and coats, but never their drinking!

TOAST   Here's a toast to a great nightclub operator—someone whose life is mostly wine, women and aspirin.

NIGHT WATCHPERSON

ROASTS   If he's a night watchman, how come he's always walking around in a daze?

She may be a night watchperson, but she certainly has a lot of daydreams!

He's a real night owl on the job, but he doesn't give a hoot about anything!

She's not afraid of her job as a night watchperson—she can sleep right through it!

BOAST   I enjoy my job as a watchperson—I actually get paid to sleep away from home!

TOAST   Let's lift a toast to a fine night watchperson—someone who never worked a day in his life!

NOTARY

ROASTS   She may call herself a notary, but others call her notorious!

The only thing really notable about him is his odd face!

If there is anything you can authenticate about her face, it's *notarize*!

With his reputation, not only shouldn't he be a notary public, he shouldn't do *anything* in public!

BOAST   I'm the best notary public in town, and I can authenticate that!

TOAST   Here's a toast to a fine notary—someone who is best known by his deeds!

NURSE

ROASTS   His specialty is waking you in the middle of a nap to take a sleeping pill!

You can easily tell she's a nurse from her *bed*pan expression!

He's a practical nurse—he ended up marrying a rich patient!

All the other nurses call her "Tonsil" because so many doctors take her out!

BOAST   I never have anything to do with bedpans—I'm the *head* nurse!

TOAST   Let's lift a toast to a great nurse—someone who thinks a dressing is something you put on a salad!

NURSERY PERSON

ROASTS   I don't know why she'd want to work in a nursery—she has enough kids at home!

Naturally, he's a nursery person—his reputation is already soiled!

She acts just like one of her hothouse flowers—always coming home potted!

He's a very lazy nursery person—always found in beds!

BOAST   I'm a very sexy nursery person—people are always getting into my plants!

TOAST   Here's a toast to a fine nursery person—someone who can always be caught with his *plants* down!

NUTRITIONIST

ROASTS   He tells you to eat what you don't want, drink what you don't like and do what you'd rather not!

She calls herself a nutritionist! Yesterday, I caught her eating lunch at a fast-food restaurant!

He's a nutritionist with his own basic food groups: candy, pies and cakes, ice cream and munchy snacks!

She takes so many vitamins, she bends the spoon when she stirs her coffee!

BOAST   As a nutritionist, I know the best way to stay in good health—don't get sick!

TOAST   Let's lift a toast to a brave nutritionist—someone who actually follows the advice he gives!

O

OBSTETRICIAN

ROASTS   You can easily tell he's an obstetrician—his conversation is filled with pregnant pauses!

She has two things in common with the stork—childbirth and the size of his bill!

Every day he works as an obstetrician, he celebrates a holiday—Labor Day!

She's way overpaid for her work—all she does is make small deliveries!

BOAST   I'm a very successful obstetrician—I make all my money on the *stork* market!

TOAST   Let's lift a toast to a great obstetrician. Nowadays, most of his patients are accident cases!

OFFICE WORKER

ROASTS   She's so terrible an office worker, the only thing she's good at filing are her nails!

He's already a month behind his work at the office, and he's only been with the company a month!

She made a great discovery at the office the other day—she found out the dictionary lists words alphabetically!

He spends so much time at the office water cooler, he's beginning to grow fungus!

BOAST   The boss says I'm a very responsible office worker— if anything goes wrong at the office, I'm responsible!

TOAST   Here's a toast to an office worker who's great at taking messages—and anything else he can get his hands on!

OIL WORKER

ROASTS   Naturally, he's an oil worker—in the Army he was a drill sergeant!

She's a dedicated oil worker—she'll go to great depths to please the company!

He went to the dentist but had no teeth problems. He said, "Drill anyway, I feel lucky!"

Naturally, she's an oil worker—everything she does is slippery!

BOAST   I like working on a drilling rig even though it means *oily* to bed and *oily* to rise!

TOAST   Let's lift a toast to the oil worker's motto: *oil's* well that ends well!

ONEIROCRITIC

ROASTS   She may be good at interpreting dreams, but she looks like a nightmare!

He's so dumb, he thinks a nightmare is a lady horse that won't work the day shift!

She has a great plan for a double night's rest—just dream that you're sleeping!

He says his wife is a real dream. Too bad, mine's actually living!

BOAST   I recommend you always wear your glasses to sleep, that way you get a better look at what you're dreaming!

TOAST   Here's a toast to a great oneirocritic. Now if only he could get himself to stop snoring!

OPTICIAN

ROASTS   He's a terrible optician—all he ever has are shattering experiences!

She has absolutely no tact with her patients—she calls them all "Four-Eyes!"

The only kind of glasses he really cares about are filled with booze!

He's so terrible an optician, he couldn't even frame a picture!

BOAST   I'm an optician with much influence, after all, I do have a lot of contacts!

TOAST   Let's lift a toast to a very prosperous optician—someone to whom a small bill is an optical illusion!

OPTOMETRIST

ROASTS   She's thinking of joining practice with a dentist—to work on eye teeth!

He's an optometrist who never uses glasses—he prefers to drink straight from the bottle!

She's so dumb, she recommended contact lenses to a patient to find his glasses!

He told a lady patient to stop wearing glasses—she wouldn't see as well, but she'd look a lot better!

BOAST   I had very bad eyesight until I was age five—then I got a haircut!

TOAST   Here's a toast to an optometrist who knows what to advise for clearer vision—weaker drinks!

ORNITHOLOGIST

ROASTS   Obviously, he's an ornithologist because his job is for the birds!

Naturally, she's an ornithologist because she's an expert at collecting bills!

You can easily tell he's an ornithologist because he's always wasting his time on some lark!

Of course, she's an ornithologist because people are always giving her the bird!

BOAST   My boss is also into ornithology because he watches me like a hawk!

TOAST   Let's lift a toast to a true ornithologist—someone who's afraid to fly!

OSTEOPATH

ROASTS   He's such a terrible osteopath, he always works his fingers to your bones!

She's such a terrible osteopath, she's always rubbing her patients the wrong way!

Naturally, he's an osteopath because he has a bone to pick with other types of doctors!

I'm not too sure about her medical qualifications. She refers to osteopathy as the lazy man's gymnastics!

BOAST   I believe in osteopathy because I feel in your bones it's the best treatment of disease!

TOAST   Let's lift a toast to a dedicated osteopath—someone who's always boned up on his profession!

P

PACKAGER

ROASTS   He's a natural packager—even as a kid, he had his hands into everything!

She's so dumb a packager, she still thinks babies are delivered by parcel post!

He's so dumb a packager, he packs everything from inside the box!

She thinks she's a qualified packager because she used to be a professional boxer!

BOAST   I'm so great at my job, even when I proposed to my wife, I fought for a package deal!

TOAST   Let's lift a toast to a great packager—someone who's living proof that little things come in small packages!

PAINTER

ROASTS   Naturally, he's a painter—people are always giving him the brush!

She's a very meticulous painter—she insists on painting by the number!

They call him an Indian painter because he always uses old paint!

He works part-time with a palm reader—for people who want their palms red!

BOAST   I enjoy my work so much, when I'm off the job I like to paint the town red!

TOAST   Here's a toast to a true painter—someone who specializes in off-color jokes!

PALM READER

ROASTS   He's so dumb, he moved to California because he heard the streets are lined with palms!

She's so dumb, she bought a bucket of paint for people who want their palms red!

He's so conceited, he's always expecting people to give him a hand!

She's such a pest of a person, really difficult to get off your hands!

BOAST   I'm a well-prepared palm reader—I always know my lines!

TOAST   Let's lift a toast to someone who knows all about hands, except how to keep them out of your pocket!

PARAMEDIC

ROASTS   Naturally, she's a paramedic—with her lousy medical training, she has to keep on the move!

The only time there's an emergency to him is when he runs out of beer in the refrigerator!

They call her a paramedic? Somebody should call *her* a paramedic!

He's so terrible a paramedic, who ever hired him needs a pair-a-glasses!

BOAST   I'm so brave a paramedic, somebody ought to pin a pair-a medals on me!

TOAST   Here's a toast to a religious paramedic—someone who just loves revival meetings!

PARKING ATTENDANT

ROASTS   There's one sure thing about this parking attendant—he always does a bang-up job!

She parks cars so close, if you give her an inch, she'll take a fender!

He has a twin who also shares the same job—they're known as the parker brothers!

She's a parking attendant who's also an opportunist—always looking for an opening!

BOAST   My job may look easy, but it's not all that it's cracked up to be!

TOAST   Let's lift a toast to an aware parking attendant—always ready to scrape you up a good deal!

PARTS SUPPLIER

ROASTS   Her big problem is letting the guys know which parts are *not* available!

He'd do a much better job supplying parts if he could just get *himself* together!

She once got kicked out of acting in a play because she forgot her part!

He's so terrible at his job, he couldn't supply a proper part for his own hair!

BOAST   I don't go out with foreign girls anymore—their parts are too hard to get!

TOAST   Here's a toast to a true parts supplier—someone whose mind is *partly* there!

PARTY PLANNER

ROASTS   He specializes in Gay-90's parties—where all the men are gay and the women are 90!

Her parties are so cheap, the water always flows like champagne!

He likes to give away door prizes at his parties. Last time he gave away six doors!

She always gives a surprise party—it's always a surprise if it's any good!

BOAST   I'm so crazy about parties, I give a going away party when I take out the garbage!

TOAST   Let's lift a toast to someone whose parties are always formal and stiff—he's formal and the guests are stiff!

PAWNBROKER

ROASTS   She inherited her money-lending profession—her ancestors were Pawnee!

He's always ready to make advances to women, regardless of their age or appearance!

She knows that you're always welcome to see her at your earliest inconvenience!

He doesn't seem to mind that he makes a living off the *flat* of the land!

BOAST   Well, I can boast one thing—my job gives me a redeeming quality!

TOAST   Here's a toast to the pawnbroker's motto: it's always darkest just before the *pawn*!

PAYROLL WORKER

ROASTS   He's in charge of the money that's approximately equal to half of what you're really worth!

When she gets through with the deductions on your pay, the only thing you have for a rainy day is a pair of galoshes!

If you earn roughly $200, when she smooths it out you have almost $26.50!

He sees so many different paychecks in his job, the other fellow's wallet always looks greener!

BOAST   I finally figured out why they call it payroll—that's the money that just rolls away!

TOAST   Let's lift a toast to the payroll worker—someone for whom when the roll is called up younder will receive his true pay!

PEDIATRICIAN

ROASTS   She always wanted to be a baby doctor. But at that early age she couldn't reach the operating table!

Obviously, he's a baby doctor—he just started teething!

When a kid swallowed a nickel, she made the parents cough up fifty dollars!

He's really a fine baby doctor but he'll be even better when he grows up!

BOAST   One of my current patients is a barber's baby—a little shaver!

TOAST   Here's a toast to a true pediatrician—someone who has to stop work once every day for a nap!

PERFUMER

ROASTS   Obviously, he's a perfumer, because his job really stinks!

She credits her success to sticking her business into other people's noses!

He thinks just because he charges more per ounce, it's better perfume!

She puts high prices on her perfume so she can make more dollars and less scents!

BOAST   I know the perfumes I make are terrific because they hold everyone *smell*bound!

TOAST   Let's lift a toast to a typical perfumer—someone who makes a lot of scents!

PERSONNEL WORKER

ROASTS   He may work in personnel, but there's one thing he doesn't have—personality!

When she heard she was in charge of employee records, she brought her phonograph to work!

As a personnel director, there's only one thing that he really hates—people!

She's good at hiring people who never make mistakes but takes orders from others who make plenty of them!

BOAST   I hire people for something I really don't believe in for myself—hard work!

TOAST   Let's lift a toast to a personnel worker who hires truly special people—some who are good for something, and some who are good for nothing!

PHARMACIST

ROASTS   She has a fine background to be a pharmacist—she used to peddle drugs!

He was forced to become a pharmacist . . . to cure himself of indigestion after his wife's cooking!

She's obviously a pharmacist—her personality is a real pill!

He's so dumb, he tells customers who forget to shake the bottle to jump up and down!

BOAST   I had to learn a foreign language to become a pharmacist. . . to read doctors' prescriptions!

TOAST   Here's a toast to a true pharmacist—someone who specializes in giving folks some of his own medicine!

PHILOSOPHER

ROASTS   As a philosopher, he always knows what to do in a situation—until it happens to him!

She's always ahead of her time with ideas, but behind time with her payments!

He's a true philosopher—he never feels badly after he makes an ass of himself!

She writes about things she doesn't understand, then makes you think they're all your fault!

BOAST   At least now I can view misfortune more calmly, so I can be unhappy more intelligently!

TOAST   Let's lift a toast to a true philosopher—someone who keeps learning more about less and less, until he finally knows everything about nothing!

PHOTO COPIER

ROASTS   If she fell into the photo copy machine, she'd undoubtedly be beside herself!

There's one thing true about his work—he always makes the same mistake at least twice!

She's so used to making copies of everything, for her next birth she wants twins!

He's so dumb, he put his girl friend in the photo copy machine so they could double date!

BOAST   I'm so cool at my job, they ought to call me a copy cat!

TOAST   Here's a toast to an enterprising photo copier—someone who duplicates his paycheck!

PHOTOGRAPHER

ROASTS   I'm not so sure he really knows too much about photography. He keeps taking his used flash bulbs back to the photo shop to exchange!

She has a figure that reminds you of a new roll of film—undeveloped!

His photographs are so bad, he should be arrested for indecent exposure!

It was only natural she should become a photographer—she's always thinking negatively!

BOAST   I really find being a terrific photographer quite easy. In fact, it's a snap!

TOAST   Let's lift a toast to the photographer—his favorite song is "Some Day My Prints Will Come!"

PHYSICAL THERAPIST

ROASTS   The only thing he's good at exercising is his right elbow at the corner bar!

The only kind of limbs she knows anything about are tree limbs!

He's so dumb, he has trouble exercising a thought!

Her most strenuous exercise is getting out of bed in the morning!

BOAST   I like developing exercises for other people just as long as *I* don't have to do any of them!

TOAST   Let's lift a toast to a true physical therapist—someone who's an expert at getting people tired!

PIANO TUNER

ROASTS   She's someone who always works for scale!

As far as an instrument to tune, the piano is his forte!

Whenever she tunes a piano, her left hand never knows what her right hand is doing!

He says he has trouble opening a piano because all the keys are inside!

BOAST   Naturally, I'm a piano tuner because I'm so grand and upright!

TOAST   Here's a toast to a fine piano tuner—too bad he doesn't know how to play one!

PILOT

ROASTS   She has a lot in common with burlesque strippers— they're both concerned with takeoffs and landings!

He's always considerate toward his passengers. He never lets them see him bring aboard his pacifier!

She's an experienced pilot. She knows no airplane ever backed into a mountain!

He always puts his craft on automatic pilot. He knows it's always safer in the back of the plane!

BOAST   I'm a class flyer all the way. I'm the only pilot I know of who has personalized airsickness bags!

TOAST   Here's to a pilot who never overdoes his job. He says he doesn't want to run it into the ground!

PLANNER

ROASTS   He has no business making other people's plans—he can't even make any of his own!

Every day before she goes to work she says the same old thing: "Well, back to the drawing board!"

Her planning comes out all the same—something either abandoned or unfinished!

His economic plans always include everything but economy!

BOAST   I know I'm a great planner. I always include a good excuse for after the plans don't work!

TOAST   Let's lift a toast to a great planner—someone who puts off until tomorrow what he has no intention of ever doing!

PLASTERER

ROASTS   Sure, she's great at her job—she has plenty of practice being plastered!

He's so dumb, he couldn't even put on a good corn plaster!

She's so dumb, she traveled to France to buy some plaster-of-Paris!

He's so lazy, you have to drive him to the wall to get him to plaster!

BOAST   I'm so crazy about my work, even when I go to the ball-park, I wrap my hot dog in a mustard plaster!

TOAST   Here's a toast to a true plasterer—someone who can really put it on thick!

PLASTIC SURGEON

ROASTS   He's so bad a plastic surgeon, he just maims to please!

She always lifts faces twice—the second time after the patient sees the bill for repairs!

He must use gunpowder to fix faces—they all look shot!

Her patients all have complexions like peaches—yellow and fuzzy!

BOAST   I once worked on a girl who had such a pretty chin I added two more!

TOAST   Let's lift a toast to a true plastic surgeon—someone who's always sticking someone else's nose into his business!

PLUMBER

ROASTS   Naturally, she's a plumber—she comes from Flushing!

If anyone thinks they'll get a fair deal from him, it's a pipe dream!

Paying her to do a good plumbing job is just like pouring money right down the drain!

Naturally, he's a plumber—everyone is always telling him to pipe down!

BOAST   I'm such a great plumber, I never leak any of my trade secrets!

TOAST   Here's a toast to an inconsistent plumber—someone whose business is always running hot and cold!

PODIATRIST

ROASTS   He provides all the needed services, and the patient *foots* all the bills!

She promised a patient that she'd have him walking in no time. She did—she took his car!

He's so dumb, he thinks a podiatrist makes house calls in a *toe* truck!

Her advice for pain in the left foot is phenomenal—walk on the *right* foot!

BOAST   I'm a podiatrist who yearns to be in the theatre—I've always wanted to be before the footlights!

TOAST   Let's lift a toast to a fine podiatrist—someone who knows that athletes have athlete's foot, and astronauts have missletoe!

POET

ROASTS   She has absolutely no business being a poet, because most poets have absolutely no business!

He tries to put a lot of fire into his verses—he should put his verses into the fire!

She's a poet with a great imagination—she imagines people will read her poems!

There's only one way his writing will be accepted by a magazine—if he writes a check for a subscription!

BOAST   I often have some really great ideas for poems, usually when I don't have a pencil!

TOAST   Here's a toast to a great poet—someone whose life is filled with many verses and a great deal more reverses!

POLICE PERSON

ROASTS   He asked to join the Swat Team—they gave him a job in the precinct office killing flies!

She's such a terrible cop, she should really quit and join the police *farce*!

His policy is to just leave burglars alone. . . so they'll become rich enough to quit!

She's such a dumb cop, she once gave out a dozen parking tickets before she found out she was at a drive-in movie!

BOAST   Not only do I know I'm a terrific cop, I'm the best that money can buy!

TOAST   Here's a toast to quite an attractive lady cop—all the guys on the force say she's great in a pinch!

POLISHER

ROASTS   He's such a terrible polisher, he can't even shine his shoes!

She may think she's a great polisher, but her culture has absolutely no polish!

Naturally, he's a polisher—he's great at shining on all his friends!

She's such a terrible polisher, she can't do anything to the finish!

BOAST   I polish everything so bright, the shine is a true reflection of my work!

TOAST   Let's lift a toast to someone who started his profession early in life—as an apple polisher!

POLITICIAN

ROASTS   Her political machine is so well-oiled, it's a wonder she has so much friction!

He's such a busy politician, he can't find any time to be honest!

She's such a terrible politician, the only time she reaches out her hand to someone is to take a bribe!

He's known in his party as a political plum—the result of careful grafting!

BOAST   My political rival has been doing a terrible job for years. Now's the time to give *me* a chance!

TOAST   Here's a toast to a typical politician—someone who is sworn into office and cussed out afterwards!

POSTAL WORKER

ROASTS   You have to watch out you don't catch anything from him—he's a carrier!

Naturally, she's a postal worker. As a kid, her favorite game was post office!

He's so dumb a postal worker, he's still trying to find the zip code for Lincoln's Gettysburg Address!

She always has such a terrible smell. She must work in the dead letter office!

BOAST   I know I'm a terrific postal worker because I always have so much zip!

TOAST   Let's lift a toast to a typical postal worker—someone whose mind has no forwarding address!

PRETZEL MAKER

ROASTS   Naturally, she's a pretzel maker—she has such a twisted mind!

Naturally, he's a pretzel maker—he has such a salty disposition!

There's only one thing that would make her life complete—to marry a beer-maker!

He's so dumb, he thinks a pretzel is only a cracker with the cramps!

BOAST   I'm so crazy about pretzel making, my favorite dance is the Twist!

TOAST   Here's a toast to a true pretzel maker—someone who only reads mystery stories with *twist* endings!

PRINCIPAL

ROASTS   He may be well-schooled in his profession, but he doesn't have a single principle!

She's been watching too much television. Now she wants everyone to start calling her "Chief!"

I wouldn't want to say it's a dog of a job being a principal, but the teachers are calling him "Prince!"

She's so dumb, she decided to vacation in Monaco this year because she heard it's a principality!

BOAST   I know that I'm a very strict principal, but I think I do a spanking good job!

TOAST   Let's lift a toast to a fine principal—someone who has the job because he's too dumb to be a teacher!

PRINTER

ROASTS   It's no wonder she's always so busy—she has so many pressing matters!

Actually, he's forced to print everything—his handwriting is terrible!

Printing for her is an old family profession—all her relatives were arrested as counterfeiters!

He's so terrible a printer, he always leaves a bad impression!

BOAST   As a printer, not only am I a person of many letters but the job is just my type!

TOAST   Here's a toast to a great printer—someone who is a person of many faces!

PROBATION OFFICER

ROASTS   He always seems to be in the doghouse with his wife, but right now he's out on probation!

She works with criminals on probation—until the next time they're caught!

He's so terrible a probation officer, the way he works with his people is a real crime!

She's so terrible a probation officer, she's the only one in the office who's on probation!

BOAST   I'm a probation officer whose conversation is very brief—all my people hate long sentences!

TOAST   Let's lift a toast to a probation officer who should watch his reputation because he's always hanging out with criminals!

PROCESS SERVER

ROASTS   She's so lazy, the only way to get her to work is to serve her a summons!

He's so terrible at his job, he couldn't even serve process cheese!

She's so terrible at her job, she couldn't even serve a tennis ball!

He thinks he works hard as a process server, but he always has to hand it to other people!

BOAST   I'm so great a process server, because I'm such a giving person!

TOAST   Here's a toast to a fine process server—someone who can easily summon up a lot of pride in his work!

PRODUCE WORKER

ROASTS   Naturally, she's a produce worker—she's always in the market for something!

Obviously, he's a produce worker because he's such a fruit!

She has a terrible reputation as a produce worker—rotten to the core!

Obviously, he's a produce worker—he drives everybody bananas!

BOAST   I know I'm a great produce worker. The boss says I'm the pick of the crop!

TOAST   Here's a toast to a great produce worker—someone who is plum crazy about his job!

PRODUCER

ROASTS   His old movies never die—they're just being shown on the "Late, Late Show!"

Her last movie was so bad that at a sneak preview, she had to sneak out!

Everybody had a good time at his last sneak preview—everybody but the audience!

Her last picture was so bad, the audience had to sit through it five times to get their money's worth!

BOAST   My next movie will be very unusual—the lovers in the story are married!

TOAST   Here's a toast to a fine producer—the only thing she can produce successfully is a fit!

PROJECTIONIST

ROASTS   With his terrible reputation, he should really project a better image of himself!

It's no wonder she's such a terrible projectionist—her whole life if out of focus!

Obviously, he's a projectionist—he's always well looped!

She's not a union projectionist yet—she hasn't passed the screen test!

BOAST   I think I should really be on the stage. Everyone says I have such good projection!

TOAST   Let's lift a toast to a true projectionist—someone who only lives in a *reel* world!

PROOFREADER

ROASTS   As a proofreader, he's one of few people who actually profits by other people's mistakes!

She's so used to her job, she made sure to proofread her marriage certificate!

He says an advantage to being a proofreader is that you learn how to write correct!

She's such a boozer, the only proof she's interested in reading is 100 proof!

BOAST   I once found a misprint that turned a hat into a cat and a baby sitter into a baby sister!

TOAST   Let's lift a toast to a great proofreader—someone who's a regular "type-righter!"

PSYCHIATRIST

ROASTS   Obviously, she's a psychiatrist—she doesn't just like her job, she's actually *crazy* about it!

He thinks he's a psychiatrist, but he's really a talent scout for a mental institution!

She had a patient who thought he was a dog, so she wouldn't let him on the couch!

He had a patient who thought he was an auto mechanic, so he told him to get *under* the couch!

BOAST   I really enjoy my job. I get to talk to beautiful oversexed women and get paid for it!

TOAST   Here's a toast to a true psychiatrist—someone whose patients all take their medicine lying down!

PSYCHIC

ROASTS   He's such a terrible psychic—what he's seeing is *un*believing!

Her boyfriend stopped seeing her because she couldn't predict she wouldn't get pregnant!

He gets all his predictions from the latest in modern day techniques—he uses a witchdoctor!

She's such a terrible psychic that she always has to bum carfare home from the racetrack!

BOAST   I know I'm a great psychic because I predicted that you'd all be here tonight!

TOAST   Let's lift a toast to a true psychic—someone who can predict every failed marriage but his own!

PSYCHOLOGIST

ROASTS   You can tell he's a psychologist—when a beautiful girl walks into a room, he watches everyone else!

She's great at telling people what everybody already knows in language that nobody understands!

His idea of psychology is to resort to talking about something else in order to distract you from the matter of attention!

She's so dumb, her kids use parental psychology on *her*!

BOAST   I know I'm a great psychologist—I've convinced everybody on staff that I'm needed!

TOAST   Let's lift a toast to a great psychologist—someone who's even managed to convince himself that he knows what he's talking about!

PUBLIC RELATIONS PERSON

ROASTS   She has great qualification for a public relations person—she hates people!

He's so dumb, the only thing that he knows public is the library!

Her idea of public relations is to convince people to think the same way she thinks!

She's so ugly, even her relations shouldn't be seen in public!

BOAST   I'm such a great public relations person, I've actually convinced a few people that the company has a good image!

TOAST   Here's a toast to a great public relations person—some-one who can straddle both sides of a question at once!

PUBLICITY PERSON

ROASTS   He not only thinks that truth is stranger than fiction, but that publicity is stranger than both of them!

Naturally, she's a publicity person—she always has a once-in-a-life-time story every day of the week!

He calls himself a publicity hound, which only means he's a breed with a big mouth and a long tale!

She provides a lot of publicity for her clients—all of it bad!

BOAST   As a publicity person, I not only act as a press agent, I sometimes have to be a *suppress* agent!

TOAST   Let's lift a toast to someone who really knows publi-city—something hard to get if you need it, easy if you don't!

PUBLISHER

ROASTS   She's a publisher who sets goals for herself. This year her goal is to learn to read!

He lost a bundle on his last big publishing effort—*War and Peace* in skywriting!

She's so dumb a publisher, she still thinks pocketbooks are ladies' purses!

He has such a terrible reputation as a publisher, they won't even allow him into the public library!

BOAST   I have a great publishing idea for printing all my pages on flypaper—for books you can't put down!

TOAST   Here's a toast to a successful publisher—someone who sells books by both their label and their libel!

Q

QUALITY CONTROL WORKER

ROASTS   He's so dumb, he rejected an entire shipment of life-savers because each one had a hole in it!

She's so bad at her job, she can't even control her temper!

He's such a terrible quality control worker, because his whole life is substandard!

Her husband obviously doesn't know quality, either—look at the woman he married!

BOAST   Obviously, I'm the perfect person for my job—judging quality takes someone of real quality!

TOAST   Let's lift a toast to someone who really knows quality—especially in his performance while asking for a raise!

QUARRY WORKER

ROASTS   She got fired from her last quarry job, because she took everything for granite!

You can easily tell he's a quarry worker because he's always stoned!

Her mother used to always rock her to sleep—with real rocks!

He's so dumb a quarry worker, he thinks a marble cake is made with real marble!

BOAST   I'm such a dedicated quarry worker, for my vacation I visited the Rock of Gibraltar!

TOAST   Here's a toast to a true quarry worker—someone whose favorite kind of music is rock!

R

RADIATION SPECIALIST

ROASTS   He's so terrible at his job, he couldn't even fix his apartment radiator!

She's so dumb, she thinks radioactivity is working as a disc jockey!

He's so dumb, he wouldn't know radioactivity from atoms!

Naturally, she works in radiation—everyone she contacts gets burned!

BOAST   Not only am I great in my job, I just radiate good looks and personality!

TOAST   Let's lift a toast to a great radiation specialist—someone whose remarks are always aglow!

RAILROAD WORKER

ROASTS   She shouldn't be a railroad worker—she rarely knows how to conduct herself!

The only thing he'd like to engineer is a big raise for himself!

She's working for the right company and should be sent out of town on a rail!

He joined the railroad by accident—he got on a car thinking it was a lunchwagon!

BOAST   I used to be a haberdasher for the railroad—I was in charge of ties!

TOAST   Here's a toast to a railroad worker who always knows when a train is gone—it leaves its tracks behind!

RANCHER

ROASTS   He once had ten thousand head of cattle on his ranch—no bodies, just the heads!

She has a chicken ranch—a place where everybody is afraid to work!

He calls his the Rainbow Ranch because all the cattle are bent on disappearing!

She's so dumb, she decided to sit on her stove so she could be at home on the range!

BOAST   My ranch is so big, I have ten sports cars to run around in. Twice a year, I send out the foreman to round them up!

TOAST   Let's lift a toast to someone who really likes his job as a rancher—it's the hard work he hates!

RANGER

ROASTS   She's so dumb, she insisted on getting a job she could do herself so she could be called the Lone Ranger!

He's so dumb, he wanted to become a forest ranger so he could tell people to go to blazes!

She's so terrible at her job, she's known as the forest's prime evil!

He's a ranger who talks so much on the telephone, his place is called the Tower of Babble!

BOAST   My job as a ranger is so vital, I'm the only person who's paid to plot fires!

TOAST   Here's a toast to a fine forest ranger—someone who is always living at his peak!

REALTOR

ROASTS   He's a realtor who specializes in fabricated homes—all built on lies!

In the last rainstorm, one of the houses she had listed changed zip codes three times!

With him describing a home, "no overhead" means a house without a roof!

When she sells you a building made with stucco, you become the "stuckee!"

BOAST   The real estate business has been so good for me, I might even decide to get a license!

TOAST   Here's a toast to the laziest realtor I know—she refuses to make house calls!

RECEPTIONIST

ROASTS   He's so terrible at his job, even his television set gets bad reception!

She's so dumb, she never goes to weddings—only the receptions!

There's only one thing he's receptive to—the idea of a raise!

She used to be a receptionist at a mortuary—always receiving some body!

BOAST   I used to work in a hothouse giving warm receptions!

TOAST   Let's lift a toast to a true receptionist—someone who never lets you see anyone!

RECORD EXECUTIVE

ROASTS   You can easily tell she's a record executive—her mouth is long playing!

Obviously, he's a record executive. He's wearing a vinyl suit!

She's so notorious for getting rid of artists off her label, she's known as a company record changer!

He's a record executive with a very unusual girl friend—she's 78-33 and 1/3-45!

BOAST   I've got a great promotional idea—a 12-inch record with an 11-inch hole, for people who hate music!

TOAST   Here's a toast to a typical record executive—someone whose mind is always on the flip side!

RECREATION WORKER

ROASTS   He has a hard time convincing people that his recreation job is hard work!

She should work on getting rid of her spare tire rather than other people's spare time!

He arranges fun things for people who enjoy playing when they really should be working!

She's such a terrible recreation worker, people go to her for a build-*down*!

BOAST   I enjoy being a recreation worker so much, I'm ashamed to tell people I do it for a living!

TOAST   Let's lift a toast to a real recreation worker—someone who on his day off *works*!

REFRIGERATION WORKER

ROASTS   She's obviously a refrigeration worker—she gives all her friends the cold shoulder!

Naturally, he's a refrigeration worker—off the job he lives in a Westinghouse!

Obviously, she's a refrigeration worker—she has all her money in frozen assets!

It's no wonder he doesn't get along with people—his job leaves them cold!

BOAST   I may be a refrigeration worker, but I don't mind being paid in cold cash!

TOAST   Here's a toast to a great refrigeration worker—someone who is one of God's *frozen* people!

RESEARCHER

ROASTS   He's a researcher—that means he's been pegged to find out things his boss is too dumb to find out!

She gets all the facts together for somebody else who gets all the credit!

As a researcher, he thinks everything turns out better in the *rear* future!

Her idea is that knowledge is acquired by looking up something else!

BOAST   Unfortunately, we've just about lost the best research source—the old-fashioned partyline!

TOAST   Let's lift a toast to a real researcher—someone who's learned that the truth is the shortest distance between facts!

RESPIRATORY THERAPIST

TOASTS   Naturally, she's a respiratory therapist—her only requirement for a man is that he be alive and breathing!

He needs his own respiratory therapist—to cure his bad breath!

She's so dedicated to her job, on Halloween she wears an oxygen mask!

Naturally, he's a respiratory therapist—he's always expelling gas!

BOAST   There's a major benefit to my job—I never have to wait in line for gas!

TOAST   Here's a toast to a typical repiratory therapist—someone who failed his breath test!

RESTAURATEUR

ROASTS   His restaurant is so crummy, even the mice there go out to eat!

The menu prices at her restaurant are so high, it takes *two* credit cards to pay the check!

He's so cheap, his restaurant is the only one in town that has a substitute for margarine!

She's such a clever restaurateur whenever they run out of chocolate pudding, she adds shoe polish to the vanilla!

BOAST   I serve delicious soup du jour at my restaurant. It's made from only the finest and freshest du jours available!

TOAST   Let's lift a toast to a true restaurateur—someone who's never had the guts to eat at his own restaurant!

ROAD WORKER

ROASTS   Naturally, she's a road worker—her life is nothing but a constant rut!

He's so dedicated to his job, he sleeps in a roadbed!

There's one thing that's always way up the road for her—a raise in pay!

He's so terrible at his job, his bad roads are the best concrete evidence!

BOAST   I'm so clever a road worker, it was my idea to blend martinis for the whole crew in a cement mixer!

TOAST   Here's a toast to a typical road worker—his wife wraps his lunch in a roadmap!

RODEO RIDER

ROASTS   Naturally, he's a rodeo rider—he can throw more bull than anyone else I know!

There's only one reason why she joined the rodeo—to corral a man!

All through the rodeo, he rides tall in the saddle—too many saddle sores!

She's such a gentle rodeo rider she rides her horse side-saddle!

BOAST   I'm only a part-time rodeo rider, off and on—usually more off than on!

TOAST   Let's lift a toast to a true rodeo rider—someone who's always ready and willing to tie one on!

ROOFER

ROASTS   She hasn't done very well as a roofer—business has been falling off lately!

He hasn't done very well as a roofer lately—there hasn't been enough overhead!

You can easily tell she's a roofer because she's always in a peak!

I think he's been working too hard as a roofer—he just came down with a case of shingles!

BOAST   I know I'm a successful roofer because I couldn't nail down a better job!

TOAST   Here's a toast to a great roofer—someone who's always got you covered!

S

SADDLEMAKER

ROASTS   You can easily tell he's a saddlemaker—he's always taking things out on people's hides!

You can easily tell she's a saddlemaker—she likes to do things on the *spur* of the moment!

We should all chip in and buy him something that's symbolic of his job—a chafing dish!

He hasn't done too well as a saddlemaker because his customers are falling off!

BOAST   Don't ever try to bargain prices with me—I never saddle for less!

TOAST   Let's lift a toast to a true saddlemaker—someone who likes to play hide and seek!

SALESPERSON

ROASTS   She's such a fast talker, she needs to have the wind taken out of her sales!

He's so pushy in his profession, he specializes in sales persistence!

She works door-to-door, finding out why people don't want to buy her product!

He's such a slick salesman, his mouth runs smoother than his car!

BOAST   I'm such a super salesperson, I could sell transistor radios in Japan!

TOAST   Here's a toast to a real salesman—he convinced his wife to marry him!

SANDBLASTER

ROASTS   He's so dumb a sandblaster, he takes dynamite with him to the beach!

She's just right for her job—she's a blasting idiot!

I don't think he likes his job—his boss always has him against the wall!

She's so dumb, for lunch she thinks she can eat the *sand which* is there!

BOAST   I have special headgear for my job. I call it my blasting cap!

TOAST   Let's lift a toast to someone who really enjoys his job—he thinks life is a blast!

SANTA CLAUS

ROASTS   She's living proof that the nicest man in the world really is a *myth*!

He has a terrible reputation as a Santa because he runs around with a bag all night!

She still believes in Santa so much, every year she hangs up her nylon stockings!

He had Mrs. Santa very upset when he told her he could only come once a year!

BOAST   Even Santa has spare time to work in his garden, so all year long for me it's hoe-hoe-hoe!

TOAST   Here's a toast to a Santa who enjoys laughing at his own jokes—in other words, he really *sleighs* himself!

SCIENTIST

ROASTS   He's always trying to prolong life so we can have more time to pay the bills we owe!

She likes to call ordinary things by such long names that you think she's talking about something else!

He's a nuclear scientist—that means he needs help to screw in a light-bulb!

She plans to work herself to death, so that she'll be remembered after she's dead!

BOAST   I'd like to leave my body to science while I'm still living—to several beautiful blonds!

TOAST   Let's lift a toast to a true scientist—someone who's able to open a child-proof bottle!

SCULPTOR

ROASTS   Obviously, she's a sculptor—when they made her, they threw both her *and* the mold away!

He may call himself a artist, but as a sculptor he doesn't cut much of a figure!

She may think she's a great sculptor, but she should really do something about her busts!

Naturally, he's a sculptor—everyone knows that he's just a chiseler!

BOAST   I treat all my subjects well—every one is put on a pedestal!

TOAST   Here's a toast to a true sculptor—someone who just keeps chipping away!

SECRETARY

ROASTS   They don't dare fire her—she's the only one in the office who understands her crazy filing system!

He's really a great secretary—he can lose anything systematically!

She was on her secretarial job only two weeks and she was a month behind in her work!

He found the most dangerous position in which to sleep—with his feet on his desk!

BOAST   I know I can't type too well but I can erase 60 words a minute!

TOAST   Here's a toast to a very efficient secretary—he hasn't missed a coffee break in five years!

SEISMOLOGIST

ROASTS   She bought land in Nevada so when California falls into the ocean she'll have beachfront property!

He thinks alcoholics make good seismologists because they're so familiar with the shakes!

He can easily predict an earthquake—whenever his mother-in-law falls out of bed!

She's so dumb, she thinks earthquakes always happen at the crack of dawn!

BOAST   I really don't get paid much as a seismologist—I only work for scale!

TOAST   Let's lift a toast to a seismologist truly dedicated to his job—he only drinks shakes!

SERVICE STATION ATTENDANT

ROASTS   He's a service station attendant—that means he specializes in off-the-highway robbery!

She's so dumb, she thinks a service station attendant has to wear pumps!

One thing's for certain—both the Arabs and their prices are getting fatter!

She's pumped so much gasoline, she named her first daughter Ethyl!

BOAST   I've got a new deal at my station—easy, long-term payments on a tank of gas!

TOAST   Let's lift a toast to a typical service station attendant—someone who is always expelling gas!

SEWER WORKER

ROASTS   She has a terrible job, but it does make a lot of *scents*!

You really have to wonder about him—everything he does is such a waste!

One thing's for sure about her job—when she says it stinks, it *really* stinks!

He's ashamed to tell people he's a sewer worker. He says he works for the underground!

BOAST   Just remember one thing—it may be sewage to you, but it's bread-and-butter to me!

TOAST   Here's a toast to a typical sewer worker—someone whose boss tells him to pipe down!

SEWING PERSON

ROASTS   He must have a very musical job—he says he only works with Singers!

Naturally, she's a sewing person—she's only interested in the *seamy* side of life!

He's quite mediocre at his job—everything he makes is only sew-sew!

She's more interested in darning her husband than his socks!

BOAST   I know I'm a very funny sewing person—at least I keep myself in stitches!

TOAST   Let's lift a toast to a typical sewing person—someone who hems and haws!

SHERIFF

ROASTS   She once worked for a guy who wore a badge with a six-pointed star—he was a Jewish Sheriff!

His idea of law and order is to round up a few beers at the corner bar!

She's such a sex-starved sheriff, she's only interested in the size of her posse!

The sheriff must have a lot of friends. I heard they want to throw him a necktie party!

BOAST   As sheriff, I believe that all persons should obey all duly constipated authorities!

TOAST   Here's a toast to a sheriff who believes in the wheels of justice—just so long as they're well-greased!

SHIPBUILDER

ROASTS   He's so dumb, he thinks shrimp boats are built for midgets!

She likes building ships—at least she's sunk a lot of money into them!

He runs his home like a ship with himself as the captain. It's too bad he married an admiral!

She's so dumb, she christened her last ship *Canasta* because it has two decks!

BOAST   I may build many large ships, but I never go overboard!

TOAST   Let's lift a toast to a great shipbuilder—someone whose ships don't sink often—each only once!

SHIPPER

ROASTS   I wouldn't want to say her transportation is ancient, but when you call to ship something he asks, "One hump or two?"

I received a shipment from him that was so late, when the packages finally arrived they had whiskers on them!

She's so dumb, she shipped a package to the President of the United States at his Gettysburg Address!

He makes so many mistakes in his work, people now call him a *slipping* agent!

BOAST   I say, don't let others ship your packages so they arrive late—let *me* do it for you!

TOAST   Here's a toast to a typical shipper—someone who sends his own Christmas packages late!

SHOEMAKER

ROASTS   If you want to see one of the top loafers, he's the one you should go to!

She's so dumb, if you're interested in a pair of alligator shoes, she'll ask what size shoe your alligator wears!

He may have a lot of shoes, but he certainly doesn't have any polish!

She has a great idea how to make your shoes look smaller—wear smaller feet!

BOAST   I know I'm a great shoemaker—I save more soles than the preacher!

TOAST   Let's lift a toast to a typical shoemaker—someone who always holds on to the last!

SHOPPER

ROASTS   She had a lot of previous experience—she used to be a shoplifter!

He's had his job so long now, his body has become shopworn!

Her mental range fits her job description—everyday she goes buy-buy!

He likes to go window shopping. Yesterday he bought five windows!

BOAST   I only have one street as my territory—every day my head is on the shopping block!

TOAST   Here's a toast to a really bright shopper—someone who picks up things fast!

SIGN PAINTER

ROASTS   He was born under a very appropriate sign: "vacancy!"

There's one thing she could do to improve her sign painting—learn to read!

He's such a terrible sign painter, even his wife is giving him the brush!

She's so dumb a sign painter, she once inquired at an archery range to paint their arrows!

BOAST   I'm a well-educated sign painter—a person of many letters!

TOAST   Let's lift a toast to someone who communicates in a special way—sign language!

SILVERSMITH

ROASTS   She may be a silversmith, but there's one thing she'll never have—polish!

He's so dedicated to his job, his favorite comedian is Phil Silvers!

She may be a silversmith, but she was born with a tin spoon in her mouth!

He's so dumb, he plated his underwear so he could call himself Longjohn Silver!

BOAST   I know I'm a great silversmith, because every job I do is sterling!

TOAST   Here's a toast to someone who's a real smooth-talker about his profession—silver-tongued at that!

SINGER

ROASTS   He's so fat a singer, you wonder how a little aria can come out of such a big area!

She gets more publicity for her low-cut gowns than for her high notes!

He's so bad a singer, he couldn't carry a tune in a wheelbarrow!

Her voice is so bad, if she had to sing for her supper, she'd starve to death!

BOAST   I may not be a very good singer, but people do like to watch my Adams's apple go up and down!

TOAST   Let's lift a toast to someone who sings a lot for charity—because nobody will offer to pay him!

SKYWRITER

ROASTS   There's only one little thing she lacks as a skywriter—knowing how to read!

Naturally, he's a skywriter—he's always got his head in the clouds!

She lost her last skywriting job because of illness—she got the hiccups!

His skywriting messages are so bad, he ought to be arrested for air pollution!

BOAST   I'm a well-respected skywriter. That's why so many people look up to me!

TOAST   Here's a toast to a true skywriter—with his job, there's always a lot of overhead!

SOCIAL WORKER

ROASTS   He's so dumb, he thinks a social worker throws church ice cream socials!

She knows very well how the other half lives—the *lower* half!

He wants his wife to know that charity begins at home, so he doesn't have to take any to the office!

She has the number one requirement for a social worker—she hates people!

BOAST   I work with the poor—the only class that thinks more about money than the rich!

TOAST   Let's lift a toast to a great social worker—someone who has little to say about what he's done, and less about what he expects to do!

SOLAR ENERGY WORKER

ROASTS   She may work in solar energy; but for all that sun, she's not at all bright!

His days are darkest when the days are darkest!

Hot weather never bothers her—she just drops the thermometer out the window and watches the temperature drop!

He's so dumb, he thinks you learn to be a solar energy worker at Sunday school!

BOAST   I'm a great solar energy worker because I always look at the bright side of things!

TOAST   Here's a toast to a great solar energy worker—someone who's afraid of getting a suntan!

SONGWRITER

ROASTS   I don't know why he's a songwriter. He's seldom calm and certainly never composed!

She can't carry a tune as a songwriter, but she sure can lift a lot of them!

He's devoted a lifetime to songwriting without becoming well-versed in it!

If you don't think her songs read well, you should hear them sung!

BOAST   I'm such a great songwriter, all my imitators died before I was born!

TOAST   Let's lift a toast to a true songwriter—someone who's better at remembering than composing!

SOUND TECHNICIAN

ROASTS   I say we should all pitch in together and get her something she can really use—a hearing aid!

In his business there's only one sound he's interested in—sound sleep!

Obviously, she's a sound technician—she always makes the most noise at a party!

He's so terrible at his work, he's neither sound of mind or body!

BOAST   Naturally, I'm successful at my business—I only make sound investments!

TOAST   Here's a toast to a typical sound technician—someone who always wears loud clothes!

SPECIAL EFFECTS PERSON

ROASTS   His best explosions come on the set when something goes wrong—explosions of temper!

She works well with miniatures because she has a mind to match!

He's such a cheap special effects man, even his house has breakaway furniture!

Naturally, she's a great special effects person—even her boy friend says she's terrific at faking it!

BOAST   I have a great idea to save money on actors in my next Western picture—use *real* bullets!

TOAST   Let's lift a toast to a true special effects person—someone who always leads a false life!

SPEECH THERAPIST

ROASTS   She's such a terrible speech therapist that she operates her own tongue like it's all thumbs!

He stutters so badly, it sounds like he's speaking broken English!

She's such a terrible speech therapist that they have her teach in sign language!

He may think he's a great speech therapist, but you can bet he never speaks a hasty word to his wife!

BOAST   I know I'm a great speech therapist because I never miss an opportunity to keep quiet!

TOAST   Here's a toast to a great speech therapist—someone who always breaks his words!

STEEL WORKER

ROASTS   He's in the iron and steel business—his wife irons and he steals!

She's so stupid, she just bought a ton of steel wool—to knit herself a stove!

Obviously, he's a terrible steel worker because he's so ill-tempered!

There's good reason why she's such an ugly steel worker—from working with so much pig iron!

BOAST   Of course, I'm a terrific steel worker—that's because I'm so refined!

TOAST   Let's lift a toast to a true steel worker—someone who is always milling around!

STEEPLE JACK

ROASTS   Since she believes in women's liberation, she wants a new job title—steeple *jacqueline*!

He's thinking of quitting his job as a steeple jack—business has been falling off!

She's so dumb, she thinks a steeple chase is a race up a steeple!

He turned down a job to climb a smokestack because he didn't want the flue!

BOAST   I know I'm a great steeple jack because people are always looking up to me!

TOAST   Here's a toast to a humanitarian steeple jack—someone who likes all kinds of steeples!

STEVEDORE

ROASTS   As a stevedore, he reminds me of Bugs Bunny—always yelling, "What's up, doc?"

Naturally, she's a stevedore—she's been carrying quite a load for some time!

He even looks like a someone who works with ships. Take a look at his stern!

Obviously, she's a stevedore—she's always concerned with her piers!

BOAST   I think being a stevedore is the best job there is to have and to hold!

TOAST   Let's lift a toast to a typical stevedore—even though he works every day, he still gets docked!

STOCKBROKER

ROASTS   She dropped a lot of money in the market today—her shopping bag broke!

The reason they call him "broker" is that after you see him, you are!

She's such a terrible broker, she's great at running your money into a shoestring!

He put half my money in toilet paper and the other half in revolving doors—I was wiped out before I could turn around!

BOAST   I'm a smart broker. I have all my money in liquid assets—booze!

TOAST   Here's a toast to a true broker—the only way he could make a killing in the market is to shoot someone!

STREET SWEEPER

ROASTS   He's a sensitive street sweeper. He quit because they put too many curbs on his work!

I don't see how she could be a great street sweeper—she doesn't even know how to clean her house!

He's so dumb, he took a broom to Ireland to join the Irish Sweepstakes!

She's so dumb, the only reason she took her job was because they told her she'd really clean up in it!

BOAST   I know I'm a great street sweeper, because the job is right up my alley!

TOAST   Let's lift a toast to a meticulous street sweeper—someone who even hand buffs them afterwards.

STRIPPER

ROASTS   Her body is so ugly that when she strips the customers yell, "Put it on, put it on!"

She has a stripper's body—without clothes, nothing looks good on her!

She has her body tattooed, but the audience complained that the pictures spoiled the view!

She's a dedicated stripper—she won't even take dressing on her salad!

BOAST   I'm really dedicated to my profession—when I play cards, I only play strip poker!

TOAST   Let's lift a toast to a great stripper—she's a girl who has everything and shows it!

STUNT PERSON

ROASTS   Naturally, he's an expert at staging bar brawls—he's in so many *real* ones!

She's great at falling through breakaway windows because she's such a *pane*!

He refuses to dive off cliffs because he doesn't like the idea of jumping to a conclusion!

She comes by crashing cars naturally because that's the way she drives her own car!

BOAST   I know I'm a great stunt person—I've got everybody fooled thinking it's hard work!

TOAST   Let's lift a toast to a true stunt person—someone willing to walk through fire and make an ash of himself!

SUPERVISOR

ROASTS   She's such a terrible supervisor, nobody has the heart to tell her she's the boss!

It's easy to tell he's the supervisor—he never does any of the work!

You can easily tell she's the supervisor—she doesn't have to be nice to everybody!

He's a big man supervisor—with a big head and a big stomach!

BOAST   I have a secret for my success: I plan my work hard, then have others do the hard work!

TOAST   Here's a toast to a true supervisor—someone who gets better men around himself, and gets around men better than himself!

SURGEON

ROASTS   Naturally, he's a surgeon—even as a kid in school he was a regular cutup!

She's such a terrible surgeon, she faints at the sight of blood—especially her own!

There's only one reason he gets by as a surgeon—he has inside information!

She's such a terrible surgeon, she has trouble cutting her own toenails!

BOAST   I'll have you know I saved several lives today—I didn't show up at the operating room!

TOAST   Let's lift a toast to a typical surgeon—people are always telling him to cut it out!

SURVEYOR

ROASTS   She's so dumb a surveyor, she thinks a quadrant is something firemen hook up their hoses to!

He's so terrible a surveyor, he never works when he doesn't feel up to measure!

She doesn't survey highways anymore—she says the job leaves her too run down!

He's got a true surveyor's marriage. His wife won't give him an inch and he has to take care of the yard!

BOAST   Naturally, I'm an honest worker. Everyone knows a surveyor has to be on the level!

TOAST   Here's a toast to a true surveyor—someone who is always plotting things!

SWIMMING POOL PERSON

ROASTS   She should be well acquainted with swimming pools—she's been in a lot of dives!

Naturally, he's a swimming pool person—he's got water on the brain!

She's so naturally dizzy, she leaves everyone she talks to swimming!

Naturally, he's a swimming pool person—he's never had a deep thought in his life because his mind is so shallow!

BOAST   I know a guy who had a hole dug in his backyard in the shape of an automobile so he could have a car pool!

TOAST   Let's lift a toast to a true swimming pool person—the only one who knows how to pull the plug!

SWORD SWALLOWER

ROASTS   I heard she's getting tired of her job. She says she's had it down to here!

He's a great sword swallower—his mother was frightened by the movie "Deep Throat!"

She claims to have gulped down a three-foot sword—anybody would find that hard to swallow!

It's easy to tell he's a sword swallower because he's such a gay blade!

BOAST   I'm such a tough sword swallower that in the mornings I gargle with razor blades!

TOAST   Here's a toast to a typical sword swallower—someone who always gets the point!

T

TAILOR

ROASTS   He just fit me for a great suit. The jacket isn't bad, but the trousers are a little loose around the armpits!

The last time I wore one of her dresses to a rummage sale, somebody tried to buy it!

I wouldn't want to say his suits are unexciting, but if he were a detective he'd be a plainclothesman!

She became a tailor quite naturally—she's very good at having fits!

BOAST   I'm really quite a funny tailor—I always keep all my customers in stitches!

TOAST   Here's a toast to a great tailor. A tribute to her is only fitting!

TALENT AGENT

ROASTS   His main client doesn't really need any talent—she's a stripper!

She'll give you a home in her heart, as long as you pay the 15 percent rent!

He gets 15 percent of everything his talent gets, except his ulcers!

She's so dumb, she booked a client in Alaska for a one-nighter. He ended up playing there for six months!

BOAST   I know I'm a great talent agent—I actually read my clients' contracts before they sign them!

TOAST   Let's lift a toast to a typical agent—someone who is always long on promises and short on memory!

TALENT SCOUT

ROASTS   She has to search for people with talent since she doesn't have any herself!

There's something else he really should be scouting—another job!

She's so terrible at her job, they even threw her out of the Girl Scouts!

He's such a terrible talent scout, he told Elvis Presley he couldn't sing!

BOAST   All the people I find are like mosquitoes—they have to pass a screen test!

TOAST   Here's a toast to a typical talent scout—someone who has a great talent for finding people with no talent!

TANNER

ROASTS   He's so terrible at his job, the only way he knows how to get color in his hides is to use suntan lotion!

She came by her job naturally—her parents were always giving her a tanning!

He's so dumb, he takes his hides to the beach to give them a tan!

Naturally, she's a tanner—she's always taking things out on people's hides!

BOAST   I'm not a prejudiced tanner—I really don't care about the color of your skin!

TOAST   Let's lift a toast to a true tanner. No matter what his health, he's always dyeing!

TATTOOER

ROASTS   Her work is so terrible, all the pictures of ships she tattoos sink!

He once tattooed a belly dancer so he could see moving pictures!

She's so dumb, she once tattooed the chest of a talent agent so he'd have a heart!

I wouldn't want to say he does a cheap tattoo job, but if you want it to last you'd better not take a bath!

BOAST   I once tattooed a very image-concious guy. He wanted to walk around with a girl on each arm!

TOAST   Here's a toast to a typical tattooer—he needles all his customers and they all get the point!

TAX PERSON

ROASTS   If you're saving up for a rainy day, he always sees to it that you get soaked!

She's a real natural for her job because she's such a taxing person!

Naturally, he's a tax person because you really have to hand it to him!

Nowadays, you have to save pennies. She and the Internal Revenue Service take care of the dollars!

BOAST   I advise people to put off buying 'till tomorrow what they can buy today, because there may be a tax on it by that time!

TOAST   Let's lift a toast to a true tax person—someone who specializes in reading fiction!

TAXIDERMIST

ROASTS   You can easily tell she's a taxidermist—she thinks she really knows her stuff!

He told his wife he wanted to keep her forever—so he stuffed her!

You can easily tell she's a taxidermist, at election time she always stuffs the ballot box!

He may be a taxidermist, but it's his wife who always beats the stuffing out of him!

BOAST   I know I'm a great taxidermist, but at Thanksgiving nobody wants me to make the stuffing!

TOAST   Here's a toast to a true taxidermist—someone who really knows if there's more than one way to skin a cat!

TEACHER

ROASTS   The kids in his class are so tough, he's the one who keeps playing hookey!

She may be a good school teacher, but away from her classroom, she doesn't have a principal!

His students are very science-minded. Even the spitballs are rocket shaped!

She works in a very old-fashioned school. The kids have to raise their hands before they can hit the teacher!

BOAST   I used to teach sex education, but the kids kept asking me for homework!

TOAST   Here's a toast to remember old school teachers: They never die, they just grade away!

TELEGRAPHER

ROASTS   No matter what his state of health, he always goes to work with a code!

She's so terrible at her job, she couldn't telegraph a thought!

He telegraphs just like he sings—off-key!

Messages are sent to her in a hurry, but she decodes them like she's asleep!

BOAST   I know I'm a great telegrapher because I'm so dashing!

TOAST   Let's lift a toast to a true telegrapher—someone who is not always operating on an open circuit!

TELEPHONE OPERATOR

ROASTS   Naturally, she's a telephone operator—she always has rings in her ears!

He can always manage to give you a wrong number out of the millions that are available!

Obviously, she's a telephone operator—because she's the talk of the town!

He may be a telephone operator, but he has terrible connections!

BOAST   I know I'm a terrific telephone operator—because I'm always plugging away!

TOAST   Here's a toast to a true telephone operator—someone who must be understood to be appreciated!

TELLER

ROASTS   Naturally, he's a teller—he belongs in a cage!

You can't get away with anything in the bank while she's around—she's a teller!

He may work in a bank but for him, there's no money in it!

She may work in a bank but she has very little interest for the customer!

BOAST   I know I'm a successful teller—every day I make piles of money!

TOAST   Let's lift a toast to a fine teller—someone who we can always bank on!

TICKET TAKER

ROASTS   Naturally, she's a ticket taker—even as a child, she was a little *tearer*!

He's such a terrible ticket taker, he's too weak to tear a ticket in half!

There's only one thing more she should know to be a good ticket taker—how to read!

He had a good reason for becoming a ticket taker: he always wanted to get into the movies!

BOAST   I'm such a great ticket taker, the boss has a special nickname for me: Stubs!

TOAST   Here's a toast to a very secretive ticket taker—someone who shreds all his work!

TILER

ROASTS   He almost killed himself the other day—he hit a golf ball in his tiled bathroom!

She thinks she's the world's fastest tiler, but then, she's always telling tile tales!

He got fired from his last tiling assignment for laying down on the job!

She had to quit her last job—she found she doesn't tile too easily!

BOAST   I know I'm a great tiler—all the chickens came to see me lay a sidewalk!

TOAST   Let's lift a toast to a true tiler—someone whose favorite book is *A* Tile *of Two Cities*!

TIMEKEEPER

ROASTS   She may be a great timekeeper, but she never knows the score!

He's such a terrible timekeeper, he's always late for work!

She's such a devious timekeeper, it's her you have to watch!

Obviously, he's a timekeeper—because he's clock-eyed!

BOAST   I'm such a dedicated timekeeper that in my spare time I raise *watch* dogs!

TOAST   Here's a toast to a true timekeeper—someone who never has time to spare!

TINSMITH

ROASTS   He makes everything out of tin. The only way to get into his house is with a can opener!

She's so dedicated to her job, instead of toilet paper she uses tin foil!

Obviously, he's a tinsmith—because he likes to *mettle* in other people's business!

She's so dedicated to her job, at Christmas she trims a tin tree. . . with tinsel!

BOAST   I'm so dedicated to my job, I'm thinking of moving to tin-pan alley!

TOAST   Let's lift a toast to a true tinsmith—someone who always likes to make a shining example!

TIRE PERSON

ROASTS   She's such a bothered tire person, because she's always worried about inflation!

He's a great example of his work, because he always carries a spare tire!

Naturally, she's a tire person—she's always treading on people!

He doesn't stock balloon tires because he thinks nobody would want to put tires on a balloon!

BOAST   I know I'm great at my job because I work hard and always tire!

TOAST   Here's a toast to a true tire person—someone who always tries to keep your hubcaps!

TABACCONIST

ROASTS   He's so dumb, he sells steel links to chain smokers!

Obviously, she sells cigarettes—she's always making an ash of herself!

There's only one thing stopping him from becoming a great tabacconist—his cigarette cough!

Sure, she's a terrific tobacconist—she's always showing her butts!

BOAST   I'm thinking of quitting my job as a tobacconist because I can't hack the hours!

TOAST   Let's lift a toast to a great tobacconist—someone who's always telling people to stuff it in their pipe and smoke it!

TOLL TAKER

ROASTS   She takes money from all the vehicular traffic, but who knows for whom the bell tolls?

He takes money on the highway all day long, but when he gets home he really gets tolled—by his wife!

She calls it highway revenue; the drivers call it highway robbery!

There's only one reason why he took his job—because he likes taking drivers!

BOAST   I really like my job, because every day I have tollhouse cookies!

TOAST   Here's a toast to a true toll taker—someone whose job takes a toll on everyone!

TOOL AND DIE MAKER

ROASTS   He may be terrible at making tools, but he'll die trying!

I wouldn't want to say her work is cheap, but a tool and your money are soon parted!

It's obvious what she does for a living, because she loves tooling around!

I wouldn't want to say he's been working a long time, but there's no tool like an old tool!

BOAST   I know I'm great at my job—because nobody can touch my tools!

TOAST   Let's lift a toast to a great tool and die maker—someone who has a lot of cutting remarks!

TOYMAKER

ROASTS   She went bankrupt selling toy boomerangs—people kept returning them!

The products he makes never sell because he spends too much time toying with his ideas!

She's got a new job working for the airlines—making toy food!

He tried to manufacture an Invisible Man Doll, but he wound it up and it disappeared!

BOAST   I have a great idea for a new Dracula Doll—you wind it up and it bites a Barbie doll in the neck!

TOAST   Here's a toast to a great toymaker—someone who enjoys his job so much because he never grew up!

TRAFFIC MANAGER

ROASTS   He's so bogged down in paperwork, the only thing he manages is a traffic jam!

She's so terrible at her job, the only thing she manages is to give everybody a headache!

When he gets back followup reports on his work, he also manages to cry a lot!

The only real traffic she can manage is when she wears a low-cut blouse at her desk!

BOAST   I manage traffic so fast, the boss is thinking of mounting a stop light on my desk!

TOAST   Let's lift a toast to a health-conscious traffic manager—someone who is always worried about his congestion!

TRAPEZE ARTIST

ROASTS   You can easily tell she's a trapeze artist, because she's such a swinger!

He may have to quit his job as a trapeze artist—he's afraid of jumping to a conclusion!

She's obviously a trapeze artist, because she's always high on something!

Obviously, he's a trapeze artist—he makes very little net pay!

BOAST   Naturally, I'm a terrific trapeze artist because I really know the ropes!

TOAST   Here's a toast to a great trapeze artist—someone who every night has to pass a bar exam!

TRAVEL AGENT

ROASTS   He's having trouble pleasing a client—she's been around the world and now wants to go someplace else!

She specializes in arranging pleasure trips—separate vacations for husbands and wives!

He met his wife at a travel agency—she was looking for a vacation and he was the last resort!

She only has to display herself if people want to look at an old ruin!

BOAST   One of my clients had a very successful trip recently— he found a parking space in every town!

TOAST   Let's lift a toast to a typical travel agent—someone whose clients usually return with brag and baggage!

TREE SURGEON

ROASTS   She used to call trees her friends until she fell out of one of her friends!

Once he broke an arm while working as a tree surgeon—he fell out of one of his patients!

She's so dumb, she thinks she can tell a dogwood tree from its bark!

He's so dumb, even though business is bad, he still wants to open a branch office.

BOAST   I know I'm a great tree surgeon, because I'll always go out on a limb for you!

TOAST   Here's a toast to a great tree surgeon—someone who can always get at that root of the problem!

TUTOR

ROASTS   He's so dumb, he's the first tutor who ever needed another tutor!

She's so dumb, she thinks a tutor plays a trumpet or a saxophone!

He'd be a great tutor if he only learned to do one thing—read!

She's a shining example of the tutor's motto: it pays to be ignorant!

BOAST   I know I'm a great tutor, because my training allows people to get along without intelligence!

TOAST   Let's lift a toast to a true tutor—someone who believes that education pays, unless you become an educator!

TV REPAIR PERSON

ROASTS   She's a lady TV repair person. That gives second meaning to the phrase "boob tube!"

He also lists himself as a psychiatrist because you call him when your TV set breaks down!

Yes, television is very educational—the whole neighborhood is sending her kids through college!

He says he has to go back again several times to each house—for reruns!

BOAST   I'm so dedicated to my work that I only eat TV dinners!

TOAST   Here's a toast to a true TV repair person—someone to whom all your money goes down the tubes!

TYPESETTER/TYPIST

ROASTS   He really shouldn't be working at his particular job, because he's not the type!

She types like magic—she can turn a cat into a hat and a baby sister into a baby sitter!

He doesn't type too well, but he can erase 30 words a minute!

If you think her typing is bad, you should see her handwriting!

BOAST   I know I'm a fast typist—I'm up to 30 mistakes a minute!

TOAST   Let's lift a toast to a typist who uses the Biblical system —"Seek and ye shall find!"

U

UNION WORKER

ROASTS   He should be well-qualified for negotiating rights—he's married!

She's really dedicated to her job—even her kids are all union made!

He's so dumb, he thinks a union rate is a wedding fee!

She used to work for the taxi union, but she couldn't hack the job!

BOAST   I think my family is taking my job too seriously—even the kids have a right to strike!

TOAST   Let's lift a toast to a long-time union worker—someone who remembers when the only strikes we had were silver and gold!

UPHOLSTERER

ROASTS   You can easily tell she's an upholsterer by the way she knocks the stuffing out of her husband!

She must come from a family of upholsterers—I heard her uncle was given the chair!

Naturally, he's an upholsterer—he comes from Davenport!

Of course she's an upholsterer—she's worn out so many loveseats!

BOAST   I know I'm a funny upholsterer because I have a lot of great material!

TOAST   Here's a toast to an untruthful upholsterer—everything he does is fabricated!

USED CAR SALES PERSON

ROASTS   Obviously, he's a used car salesman. He specializes in cars that are in no way what they used to be!

Buying from her is pure truth that it's hard to drive a bargain!

Obviously, he's a used car salesman—his vehicles are rarely what they're jacked up to be!

She's a notorious used car sales person—all her autos are in first crash condition!

BOAST   My used cars will give you absolutely no trouble—if you're the first one to use them!

TOAST   Let's lift a toast to a typical used car sales person—someone whose product some people ride while others deride!

UTILITY WORKER

ROASTS   Obviously, she works for a utility company because she's such a *light* eater!

I'll give you a hint what utility company he works for—his job is a real gas!

I don't see how she could get a job with the power company—she can't even screw in a lightbulb!

He's so difficult to get any work out of, he's really a *futility* worker!

BOAST   There's only one reason I work with the utility company—because I have so much power!

TOAST   Here's a toast to a loyal utility worker—someone who's a real electric fan!

V

VENDING MACHINE WORKER

ROASTS   His vending machines serve such bad food, they've all been condemned by the Board of Health!

She's so cheap, dinner guests at her house have to buy food out of vending machines!

You don't have to travel all the way to Las Vegas to gamble money in a machine—just put some in one of his!

I put money in one of her machines for some hot chocolate. All I got was a candy bar and a match!

BOAST   If you lose money in one of my machines, don't worry about it. That's just my tip!

TOAST   Let's lift a toast to a typical vending machine worker—someone who is always grateful for change!

VENTRILOQUIST

ROASTS   She's such a terrible ventriloquist, the only thing she can throw is a lot of bull!

Obviously, he's a ventriloquist—even without a dummy he talks to himself!

She's such a simple-minded ventriloquist, it's hard to figure out which one is the dummy!

As a ventriloquist, he really has hidden talents. Someday maybe he'll find them!

BOAST   My girlfriends like the way my lips move—all over their bodies!

TOAST   Here's a toast to a typical ventriloquist—someone whose lips move even when he isn't saying anything!

VETERINARIAN

ROASTS   He must be a veterinarian—I've seen him go out with some real dogs!

She must be a veterinarian—that explains why she's so catty!

Obviously, he specializes in treating ducks—that's why they call him a *quack* doctor!

She's so anxious to get married, that's why she took up animal husbandry!

BOAST   My girlfriends know I'm a great veterinarian because they think I'm such an animal!

TOAST   Let's lift a toast to a true veterinarian—someone who leads a dog's life!

W

WAITER/WAITRESS

ROASTS   The only time he served hot food was when the restaurant burned down!

She has very polite customers. The only thing they ask her to bring them is a smaller check!

He's such a bad waiter, when you eat alphabet soup, he reads over your shoulders!

She once had a customer who was so picky, he sent back the ice cream because it was too cold!

BOAST   I've had a lot of waiting experience. Once I worked in an insane asylum—serving soup to nuts!

TOAST   Here's a toast to a tip-top waiter—if you don't tip him, he blows his top!

WALLPAPERER

ROASTS   He's always complaining about his job because his boss has him against the wall!

She's well qualified for her job because she's such a wallflower!

He's so dumb at his job, he moved to New York City so he could paper Wall Street!

She got fired from her last job because all her comments were off the wall!

BOAST   I'm working on getting a contract that'll make me rich— papering the Great Wall of China!

TOAST   Let's lift a toast to a great wallpaperer—someone who really sticks to his work!

WARDEN

ROASTS   It's no wonder she's a warden—so many people warned her she'd end up behind bars!

Obviously, he's a warden because he makes his living by his pen!

She's such a terrible warden, the work she does is positively criminal!

You can easily tell he's a warden—he handles a lot of men with many convictions!

BOAST   I'm a very articulate warden because I specialize in long sentences!

TOAST   Here's a toast to a typical warden—someone who really hates to see you go!

WAREHOUSE PERSON

ROASTS   He makes a perfect warehouse person—because his brains are in permanent storage!

She's so terrible working in a warehouse, she'd do much better working in another kind of house!

He's so bad a warehouse person, he should take better inventory of his job!

She got fired from working at a supermarket warehouse for putting all her eggs in one basket!

BOAST   I really enjoy running a warehouse—people put a lot of stock in what I say!

TOAST   Let's lift a toast to an energetic warehouse person— he just took his forklift in for a thousand-mile checkup!

WATCH REPAIR PERSON

ROASTS   Obviously, she's a watch repair person, because she has a tic!

Obviously, he's a watch person because he has a lot of time on his hands!

Her calendar watches go so fast, they get 14 days in a week!

He thinks he's in the watch business—somebody else does the work while he watches!

BOAST   My watch repair business is so successful, that's why I'm always working overtime!

TOAST   Here's a toast to a great watch repair person—someone who's yours, mine and hours!

WEATHER PERSON

ROASTS   He knows his wife listens to his weather reports—whenever he calls home, she says the coast is clear!

Even as a co-ed in meteorological school, the boys could always take one look in her eyes and tell whether!

If he doesn't start giving more accurate weather predictions, his job future may be cloudy!

She always takes her work home with her. Maybe that's why her marriage is so stormy!

BOAST   I just received the latest Mexican weather report—chili today and hot tamale!

TOAST   Let's lift a toast to a confident weather person—he quits his job whenever the weather doesn't agree with him!

WEAVER

ROASTS   He gets paid for walking drunk down city streets—he's a professional weaver!

She got a ticket while operating a loom in her car—for weaving in and out of traffic!

He cheated a Jackson loom operator—it was the first time anybody was arrested for crossing the Mississippi weaver!

She thinks she's a great weaver, but there's not a thread of truth to it!

BOAST   I know I'm a great weaver—because I'm always spinning terrific yarns!

TOAST   Let's lift a toast to someone who took a long time learning his job—we thought he'd never weave!

WELDER

ROASTS   Naturally, she's a welder—she's always carrying a torch for someone!

He's so dumb, he taught his dog how to do his work so he could *spot* weld!

She's so dumb, she sent a sick co-worker a "get-*weld*" card!

Naturally, he's a welder—if you follow him around at night, you can see he knows all about joints!

BOAST   I think my wife would also make a great welder because she's always putting the heat on me!

TOAST   Here's a toast to a dedicated welder—someone who on Halloween always wears his welder's mask!

WIG MAKER

ROASTS   His workers know he's in a bad disposition whenever they see him wearing his hairpiece upside down. That means he's flipped his wig!

One of her customers was an American Indian who set his hairpiece on fire. He wanted to keep his wig-*wam*!

His wigs are so terrible looking, most of his customers keep them under their hat!

Naturally, she's a wig maker, because she has a lot of bills *to pay*!

BOAST   I'm a truly dedicated wig maker—even my car has a convertible top!

TOAST   Let's lift a toast to a typical wig maker—someone whose customers fool themselves into believing they can fool others!

WINDOW DRESSER

ROASTS   She's so dumb a window dresser, she just pinned up a giant bra and a blouse to the window!

He's so modest in his work, he puts blindfolds on the male window dummies while he changes the female ones!

Naturally, she's a window dresser—all the men she goes out with are dummies!

He's so dumb, when a customer asked, "May I try on that dress in the window?" he let her try it on in the window!

BOAST   I know I'm a great window dresser—because it's never a *pain* to admire my work!

TOAST   Here's a toast to a typical window dresser—someone who at home never pulls down the blinds!

WINDOW WASHER

ROASTS   He has a terrible habit that may get him killed some day—he always steps back to admire his work!

Naturally, she's a window washer—she's always had to sponge for a living!

Naturally, he's a window washer—anybody can see right through him!

You can easily tell she's a window washer, because she's such a *pane*!

BOAST   I really enjoy working as a window washer—it keeps me from being arrested as a Peeping Tom!

TOAST   Let's lift a toast to a great window washer—someone who is a true reflection of his work!

WINEMAKER

ROASTS   She really qualifies to be an expert winemaker—she's a certified alcoholic!

He selected the wine for us this evening. Can anyone tell me, is four o'clock a good vintage?

You can easily tell what she does for a living, because she's always *whining*!

He likes to seduce women with champagne because he finds it's the wine of least resistance!

BOAST   I just invented the electric corkscrew—it's for the wino who has everything!

TOAST   Here's a toast to a typical winemaker—someone who hears everything through the grapevine!

WOODWORKER

ROASTS   He's so cheap, he's the guy who makes all the wooden nickels!

She fits right into her job because her personality is so wooden!

It's easy to tell what his job is because he has a woodpecker!

I wouldn't want to say her woodwork is terrible, but it's the worst work she ever *saw*!

BOAST   Woodworking has always been quite easy for me, in fact, it's as easy as sawing off a log!

TOAST   Let's lift a toast to a typical woodworker—someone who daily has to face a lot of *knotty* problems!

WRAPPER

ROASTS   She's so terrible at her work, the only thing she deserves is a good *wrap* in the mouth!

He's so dumb, he wants to move to Beverly Hills because he thinks they gift wrap the garbage!

Naturally, she was well qualified for her job—she's always *rapping* people!

He had his girlfriend thrown in jail, but she wouldn't take the *wrap*!

BOAST   I know I'm a great wrapper—the bosses offered me a package deal!

TOAST   Here's a toast to a typical wrapper—someone whose business is always folding!

WRECKER

ROASTS   It's easy to tell what he does for a living because he looks a wreck!

Obviously, she's a wrecker—all you have to do is take a look at her house!

Obviously, he's a wrecker—his favorite sport is Destruction Derby!

Her favorite job is to break up happy families—as a home wrecker!

BOAST   I really enjoy my job—I always feel like a wreck!

TOAST   Let's lift a toast to a true wrecker—someone who's always smashing!

WRESTLER

ROASTS   She may have to quit her job as a professional wrestler— she can no longer afford the acting lessons!

Obviously, he's a wrestler—he always has his ear to the ground!

She's a very frustrated wrestler. Her psychiatrist told her to get a hold of herself!

He's obviously a wrestler, because he's always trying to make other people's ends meet!

BOAST   I know I'm a great wrestler because nobody can come to grips with me!

TOAST   Here's a toast to a wrestler who's also a great artist— he should be, he spends most of his life on canvas!

X

X-RAY TECHNICIAN

ROASTS   As an X-ray technician, he has his own definition of his job: belly-vision!

She used to go out with another X-ray technician, but she didn't see anything in him!

He always has the same answer to any of his patient's requests— "I'll look into it!"

She's so terrible at her job, she's anything but *X*-acting!

BOAST   I'm only an X-ray technician for one reason—so I can see through the day!

TOAST   Let's lift a toast to a typical X-ray technician—someone who always has negative thoughts!

XYLOPHONIST

ROASTS   She has a real gift for playing the xylophone. Now if only they'd give her one for stopping!

He's a very superstitious xylophonist because he's always knocking on wood!

The xylophone is very difficult for her to play—she's always trying to hammer a tune!

He's so dumb, he thinks a xylophone is something you call a *xylo* on!

BOAST   I keep my xylophone in my refrigerator because I like to play it cool!

TOAST   Here's a toast to a xylophonist who likes to play wooden instruments. Well, he certainly has the head for it!

Y

YACHT PERSON

ROASTS   He's so dumb, he says he never wanted a job on a yacht, because he'd rather sail a boat!

She's so terrible at her job, she really *yacht* to do something else!

He ought to be good on a yacht, even off the job he's always cruising!

She may sail a pleasure craft, but sailing with her is no pleasure!

BOAST I really enjoy my job because there's *yachting* else I'd rather do!

TOAST Let's lift a toast to someone who really knows what a yacht is—a floating debt!

YARDAGE WORKER

ROASTS Obviously, she's a yardage worker. She's only interested in material things!

Naturally, he's a yardage worker. He's always fabricating things!

Obviously, she's a yardage worker because you can't give her an inch!

He's so high and mighty about his job, he calls himself a man of the cloth!

BOAST I know I'm a great yardage worker because I do everything in good measure!

TOAST Here's a toast to a typical yardage worker—someone who always measures up to his work!

Z

ZIPPER REPAIRER

ROASTS Obviously, he's a zipper repairer, because his life has a lot of ups and downs!

She's obviously a zipper repairer, because she's always getting herself caught in something!

Obviously, he's a zipper repairer—he was just arrested for bombing a button factory!

Her job gave her a bad reputation. You might say zippers are her undoing!

BOAST   I'm so great at my job, I also work part-time for the post office fixing zip codes!

TOAST   Let's lift a toast to a great zipper repairer—someone with a job to really sink his teeth into!

ZOOKEEPER

ROASTS   She has more trouble controlling the wild children than the wild animals!

What he does is absolutely criminal—he puts animals behind bars!

Every time she goes to the zoo, she has to buy two tickets—one to get in and one to get out!

She's so dumb, during the holidays, she ordered some Christmas seals!

BOAST   I'm so famous for my work, they're going to put my name in "Who's Zoo!"

TOAST   Here's a toast to a typical zookeeper—someone who wants to work near his relatives!

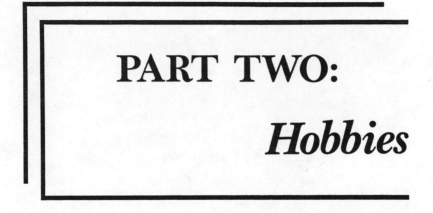

PART TWO:

Hobbies

A

ARCHERY

ROASTS   You can easily tell his hobby is archery—because he wears Arrow shirts!

She's so terrible at archery, her target never gets the point!

He's so dangerous on the archery field, everyone around him quivers!

She's so man-crazy, she can't take archery seriously—she's only interested in her *beaus*!

BOAST   I know I'm addicted to archery—whenever I hear the William Tell Overture, I *don't* think of The Lone Ranger!

TOAST   Let's lift a toast to a devoted archer—whenever he's at the movies, he cheers for the Indians!

ASTROLOGY

ROASTS   She really digs astrology—she was born under the sign "vacancy!"

He was born under the sign of Leo the lion—his mother was at an M-G-M movie at the time!

Her life has been so unlucky that lately she looks up her daily *horror*-scope!

He sees the most stars after he comes home late at night—from his wife!

BOAST   I know that many people think their lives are ruled by the planets, but most men are ruled by their wives!

TOAST   Here's a toast to a true astrology buff—someone whose head is always in the stars!

B

BADMINTON

ROASTS   Naturally, his hobby is badminton because he's always giving people the bird!

She doesn't care how much she cheats playing badminton, just so she gets the net results!

I don't think he knows too much about badminton, the other day, he nearly killed himself trying to jump over the net!

She's so terrible at playing the game, badminton is just not her racket!

BOAST   I'm so terrific at badminton, I always have my day in court!

TOAST   Let's lift a toast to a great badminton player—someone who can always beat the tailfeathers off his opponent!

BALLET

ROASTS   Actually, he's a toe dancer—because he keeps stepping on other people's toes!

One time she got so carried away while doing a pirouette, she screwed herself into the ground!

He may have to give up ballet—he's getting too big for his tutu!

She actually started ballet by accident—when somebody gave her a hot-foot!

BOAST   There's really only one reason I like ballet so much—it keeps me on my toes!

TOAST   Let's lift a toast to a great ballet dancer—someone whose performances are *too-too* much!

BASEBALL

ROASTS   He decided he liked baseball because you don't need a college education to play on a team!

She may like to play baseball, but the guys can't get to first base with her!

He plays baseball—a business he knows can't thrive without strikes!

She's such a terrible baseball player—she wouldn't hit a fly!

BOAST   I know I'm a terrific athlete—all the girls want to have a ball with me, but I'd rather play the field!

TOAST   Here's a toast to a gal we should call "Baseball"—because she won't play the game without a diamond!

BASKETBALL

ROASTS   Yesterday, she got a good tip from her basketball coach—take up chess!

He's so dumb a basketball player, he brought his pet duck to the game to play the *foul* line!

She's so dumb at the game, she'd do better with a *shopping* basket!

He's such a sloppy basketball player, when he dribbles on the court he *really* dribbles on the court!

BOAST   I know I'm a great basketball player—I always try to put all my balls in one basket!

TOAST   Here's a toast to a very legal-minded basketball player—someone who always wants to go to court!

BIKING

ROASTS   He's the only person I know who drinks while he bicycles—because he never could *handle bars*!

She's so dumb, she took up bicycling because she always wanted to be a pedlar!

As a youngster, he gave up bicycling early—he wanted to get away from his *spokes*!

She's so fat, the only way she could go biking is on a bicycle built for six!

BOAST   I have a terrific idea to promote long endurance biking—bicycles with no seats!

TOAST   Let's lift a toast to a dedicated biker—he's thinking of growing a *handlebar* moustache!

BIRDWATCHING

ROASTS   She found out birdwatching can be a messy hobby—especially if the bird spots you first!

He may call it birdwatching, but he's really looking for an easy nestegg!

She's so crazy about her hobby, at Thanksgiving she'd rather watch the bird than eat it!

He's so crazy about birdwatching, he sends fan letters to the NBC peacock!

BOAST   There's only one reason I took up birdwatching—because it fits the bill!

TOAST   Here's a toast to the true birdwatcher—someone who enjoys watching *fowl* play!

BOARD GAMES

ROASTS   He sometimes gets so mad playing checkers, when he jumps his opponent he really jumps his opponent!

It's very difficult playing chess with her because she never plays on the square!

He's so dumb, he won't play chess because he heard it takes four knights to play a game!

She won't play chess, because she doesn't want to get caught with her pawns down!

BOAST   I'm so rich, I play Howard Hughes Monopoly—using real hotels!

TOAST   Let's lift a toast to someone who's famous for playing board games—you might say he's had a checkered career!

BOWLING

ROASTS   He likes bowling because it gets him off the streets and into the alley!

She called hers a bowling alley marriage because that's where she and her husband split!

He doesn't like to take his wife to the alley—he only wants one bowling bag there at a time!

She played so well with her new bowling ball last night she might even decide to get some holes drilled in it!

BOAST   I know I'm a terrific bowler. . . why else would they call me pin head?

TOAST   Here's to a fellow who's crazy about bowling—he's always got his mind in the gutter!

BULLFIGHTING

ROASTS   He has a lot more success throwing the bull than fighting it!

She's very cowardly at her hobby—she spends most of her time fighting to get out of the ring!

He should be very good at his hobby—as a kid he was always fighting the school bully!

She may soon get into trouble with her hobby—she's always grabbing the bull by the horns!

BOAST   I'm so dedicated to my hobby, my house is guarded by a bulldog!

TOAST   Let's lift a toast to a true bullfighter—someone who can hardly wait to get in the ring, it's difficult to *pick a door*!

BUTTERFLY HUNTING

ROASTS   Obviously, she's a butterfly hunter—that's why she's always in such a flap!

He's a very anxious butterfly hunter because he's always worried about his *net* worth!

Obviously, she's a butterfly hunter—because she's such a fluttery person!

He reminds me of one of his butterflies—a worm that turned!

BOAST   I'm so crazy about butterflies, I'm going to sell my house and move into a *cocoon*-dominium!

TOAST   Here's a toast to someone truly dedicated to his hobby—his favorite swimming stroke is the butterfly!

C

CAR RACING

ROASTS   He's so terrible at car racing, he really *auto* be doing something else!

Naturally, her hobby is car racing—because she's really such a drag!

Of course, he likes speeding cars—everyone knows he's a racist!

She has such a terrible reputation in a car—more the back seat than the front!

BOAST   I'm so anxious to race cars—I'm always open to a bit of *auto* suggestion!

TOAST   Let's lift a toast to a typical car racer—someone who is always trying to horn in on other drivers!

CARDS

ROASTS   She has her own card rules she says she learned in England—London Bridge!

He knows both love and playing cards can be fun—depending on the hand you're holding!

She's very unlucky playing blackjack. But anyone can tell you she'll never see 21 again!

His friends can tell you about his card playing ability. They keep saying he doesn't have a full deck!

BOAST   I don't want to brag about being a card shark, but my friends call me "Jaws!"

TOAST   Here's a toast to a woman who compares her husband to an old deck of cards—both are hard to deal with!

CERAMICS

ROASTS   Naturally, she's into ceramics—because she's a real *crackpot*!

He's absolutely terrible at ceramics, because everything he does comes out half-baked!

Naturally, she's into ceramics—she really has the pot for it!

You can easily tell he's into ceramics—one look at him and you can tell he's gone to pot!

BOAST   I have a very conservative hobby—I'd rather make a pot than smoke it!

TOAST   Here's a toast to someone who is really into ceramics— a person with hands of clay!

CHESS

ROASTS   Obviously, his favorite game is chess—because he's always trying to get the jump on someone!

She's a very jealous chess player—she's always wanting to check her mate!

Obviously, his favorite game is chess—because he's always anxious to have a good knight!

She's so dumb, she thinks she can play chess because she's had such a checkered career!

BOAST   I'm a very honest chess player—I always play the game on the square!

TOAST   Let's lift a toast to a true chess player—someone who should never be caught with his *pawns* down!

COINS

ROASTS   She's so dumb, someone asked her if she was a numismatist and she said, "No, I collect coins!"

He's a very optimistic coin collector because he's always looking for change!

Obviously, she's a coin collector because she's always going through her couch for loose change!

His girl friend is also a numismatist. You might say she's his *coined* of gal!

BOAST   You know I didn't really want to become a numismatist—I was coined into it!

TOAST   Let's lift a toast to a true coin collector—someone who has all kinds of money!

COLLECTING

ROASTS   There's really only one thing he's good at collecting—dust!

She's really good at collecting one thing—unemployment checks!

Obviously, he's a collector—that's the way he makes all his phone calls—collect!

She's so badly in debt, collecting for her is not just a hobby, it's a pursuit!

BOAST   I'm so into my hobby, at church I'm always the one they ask to take the collection!

TOAST   Here's a toast to a true collector—someone who gathers so many different things, he can't remember what he's collecting!

COOKING

ROASTS   She's so bad a cook, she boils Green Stamps to make pea soup!

Obviously, he's into cooking because he's always in such a stir!

She's such a terrible cook—all her ideas come out half-baked!

He's such a terrible cook that the people he serves pray both before and after a meal!

BOAST   I have an easy way to make an eight-course meal: bake a seven-layer cake and serve it with coffee!

TOAST   Here's a toast to a cook who knows how to keep your food bills down—use a heavier paperweight!

CROQUET

ROASTS   He plays such a nervous game, people say he plays "chicken" croquet!

She plays such a mean game of croquet, there's nobody more *wicket*!

You've heard of a wooden leg—he's a guy who has wooden balls!

She's so crazy about croquet, she'd rather play on grass than smoke it!

BOAST   I enjoy playing solitaire croquet because "I vant to be a lawn!"

TOAST   Let's lift a toast to a dedicated croquet player—someone to whom nothing else *mallets*!

D

DANCING

ROASTS   His favorite disco is a place called "Jaws"—it costs an arm and a leg to get in there!

She may dance lightly on her feet, but not on her partner's!

He usually starts dancing on the wrong foot—his partner's!

She really wanted to be a bubble dancer but her mother said, "No soap!"

BOAST   When I dance, my feet never touch the floor—I wear shoes!

TOAST   Here's a toast to a guy who dances a terrific tango—no matter what the band is playing!

DRUMS

ROASTS   He's so dumb, he broke into his drum to see what was making all the noise!

She's so dumb, she put her drums in the refrigerator to play a cool beat!

He's so dumb, he hits his head against his drums so he can play them by ear!

She's her own manager—that's why she's always trying to drum up new business!

BOAST   I know I'm a great drummer because my playing can't be beat!

TOAST   Let's lift a toast to a true drummer—whenever he's at dinner, he reaches for the drumstick!

E

EXERCISE

ROASTS   There's one basic exercise she needs badly—pushing herself away from the dinner table!

He's so terrible at his hobby, he gets pooped exercising a thought!

She's so lazy, the only exercise she ever gets is rolling out of bed!

He has a special mental exercise—jumping to conclusions!

BOAST   I exercise a great deal to keep in shape—so much so that even my muscles have muscles!

TOAST   Here's a toast to a true exercise nut—someone who works hard convincing himself that exercise isn't work!

F

FENCING

ROASTS   He's so crazy about fencing, his favorite food is swordfish!

She's so dumb at fencing, she has to keep going back to class for pointers!

He's so dumb, he took a class in fencing to learn how to build something around the house!

She's undecided about swordfighting, but she doesn't want to straddle the fence!

BOAST   I'm so terrific at fencing, my opponents always get the point!

TOAST   Let's lift a toast to a real macho swordsman—he's anything but a gay blade!

FISHING

ROASTS   When she goes fishing, all she gets is a sunburn, poison ivy and mosquito bites!

He likes to go fishing—other people call it just drowning worms!

When she goes fishing, there's a worm on one end of the pole and a fool on the other!

He's only an amateur fisherman, but he can tell lies as big as a professional!

BOAST   I'm a very reasonable fisherman, because I have a *bait* and see attitude!

TOAST   Here's a toast to a typical fisherman—every time he talks about the one that got away, it grows another foot!

FLOWER ARRANGING

ROASTS   His flower arrangements are so terrible, even the bees won't go near them!

She's well qualified for her hobby, since she's such a wallflower!

He'd like to arrange some flowers for the woman he loves, but his wife would rearrange his face!

Her flower arranging is so terrible, somebody ought to nip that hobby in the bud!

BOAST   I like all kinds of flowers—wild, tame and cauli!

TOAST   Let's lift a toast to someone who arranges lazy flowers— because he always finds them in beds!

FLYING

ROASTS   She had to give up flying—the long trip to the airport made her car-sick!

He's such a terrible flyer, he gets sick just licking an airmail stamp!

The last time she took me up flying, the plane had engine trouble and she asked me to get out and push!

He had very early flying experience—when he was just a kid, he fell out a window!

BOAST   I just flew in from New York, folks—boy, are my arms tired!

TOAST   Here's a toast to a true flyer—someone who gets dizzy just looking at an airline ticket!

FOOTBALL

ROASTS   He's so stupid, he got into football by accident—somebody asked if he'd like to play and he said, "I'll pass!"

Everyone knows why she's into football—all the guys say she's great in a huddle!

He did something impossible while playing football the other day—he ran around his own end!

She's got quite a reputation in football—as the gal who took on the entire male team!

BOAST   I learned to play football at barber college but I kept getting penalized for clipping!

TOAST   Let's lift a toast to a true football buff—it's the only game he wants to tackle!

G

GAMBLING

ROASTS . She's so sure she can quit gambling, she's willing to lay anyone five to one odds on it!

He's so unlucky at gambling, he put a dime in a Las Vegas parking meter and lost his car!

She was sure lucky in Las Vegas on her last trip—she forgot her wallet!

He finally found an easy way to beat the slot machines in Las Vegas —with a sledge hammer!

BOAST   I did great the last time I went to Las Vegas—I arrived in a six thousand-dollar car, and left on a 30 thousand-dollar bus!

TOAST   Here's a toast to a true gambler—someone who refuses to work today because he expects to win at the races tomorrow!

GARAGE SALES

ROASTS   He just loves going to garage sales—last weekend he bought three garages!

She bought a desk at a garage sale that she swears once belonged to Benjamin Franklin. . . it still has Franklin's name carved in the Formica!

He knows just what to do when he's sitting around, down in the dumps—have a yard sale!

She eventually had her own garage sale—she had to, in order to find her car!

BOAST   I made so much money at my last garage sale, I was able to buy what I always wanted—a bigger garage!

TOAST   Let's lift a toast to a real garage sale nut—someone who buys something he doesn't want, sold at a price low enough to make him want it!

GARDENING

ROASTS She's so dumb a gardener, she sprinkled grass seed in her hair and said, "I want to be a *lawn*!"

He thinks he's such a great gardener, he just makes his own bed and has to lie about it!

Her gardening is so terrible, she's disproof that man reaps what he sows!

He's such a terrible gardener, his green thumb turned blue!

BOAST The reason I'm such a terrific gardener is because I'm such a down-to-earth fellow!

TOAST Here's a toast to a great gardener who thinks he's Santa Claus—every day it's hoe, hoe, hoe!

GEM COLLECTING

ROASTS I don't know what business he has gem collecting—he certainly doesn't have any polish!

Naturally, her hobby is gem collecting because she's always stoned!

He's thinking of expanding his hobby—he now wants to collect gems and *jellies*!

If she really thinks she collects fine gems, she should take another good look at her husband!

BOAST   The reason I'm into gem collecting is because I have so many great facets!

TOAST   Let's lift a toast to a great gem collector—someone who's not only precious but a real jewel!

GENEALOGY

ROASTS   She sent so much time and trouble looking up her family tree, only to find out she's a sap!

He traced his own family history only to find out that they were all better than himself!

She found out what part of the family tree she comes from—the shady side!

He found out the members of his own family tree are better off dead than alive!

BOAST   There's one thing I found out about the typical family tree—the best part of it is always underground!

TOAST   Here's a toast to someone who's really into genealogy—he's only trying to make a better name for himself!

GOLF

ROASTS   He claims it's no sin to play golf on Sunday. The way he plays, it's a crime!

Her golf is really improving—she's missing the ball much closer than she used to!

He wears two pair of pants when he plays golf—in case he gets a hole in one!

I don't want to accuse her of cheating, but she once had a hole-in-one and put herself down for a zero!

BOAST   I only play golf so much because of my doctor. He advised me to take plenty of iron every day!

TOAST   Let's lift a toast to a golfer who once missed a spectacular hole-in-one—by only five strokes!

GUITAR

ROASTS   He's been having a lot of trouble with his guitar lately—people keep hitting him over his head with it!

She's such a terrible guitar player, the only thing she can pick well is her teeth!

Naturally, he plays the guitar as a hobby—he's great at anything that has strings attached!

She specialized in go-go music—when she starts to play the guitar, people tell her to "Go, go!"

BOAST   I don't have on any underwear when I play the electric guitar because you have to watch out for shorts!

TOAST   Let's lift a toast to a typical guitarist—someone who's always fretting!

GYMNASTICS

ROASTS   You can easily tell she's a gymnast because she wears both spring and fall clothing at the same time!

Naturally, he's a gymnast—he has a lot of practice getting in and out of his small sports car!

She's quite naturally a gymnast, because she's always wrapped up in herself!

Obviously, he's a gymnast, because he's always horsing around!

BOAST   I'm both a great gymnast and a great friend, because I'll easily bend over backward for you!

TOAST   Here's a toast to a true gymnast—someone who has a great bent for acrobatics!

H

HANG GLIDING

ROASTS   He had to give up his hobby of hang gliding—he was afraid of jumping to a conclusion!

She had to give up her hobby of hang gliding because she couldn't get the hang of it!

His wife made him give up hang gliding. She couldn't stand the people he was hanging around with!

Naturally, her hobby is hang gliding, because people are always telling her to go fly a kite!

BOAST   Naturally, I'm great at hang gliding—because for me it's just a breeze!

TOAST   Let's lift a toast to a person who comes by hang gliding naturally—because he always has a lot of wind!

HEALTH FOOD

ROASTS   She's such a health food nut, she thinks a grape is wine in pill form!

He drinks so much to other people's health, he doesn't have any himself!

She gave up eating diet food—because she became bored of health!

He says the only way to keep your health is to eat what you don't want, drink what you don't like and do what you'd rather not!

BOAST   I'm so healthy, if everyone ate like I do, the people who make "Get Well" cards would go out of business!

TOAST   Here's a toast to someone who eats so much vitamins and health food, everytime he sneezes he cures someone!

HI-FI/STEREO EQUIPMENT

ROASTS   He's so terrible at putting his stereo equipment together, his woofers tweet and his tweeters woof!

Naturally, she's terrible with stereo equipment because she's never had any experience with fidelity!

Obviously, he has great stereo equipment—because nobody can talk over it!

She now has in her house the loudest speaker you ever heard—her mother-in-law!

BOAST   I know I have great stereo equipment because everyone who listens to it says it's such a blast!

TOAST   Let's lift a toast to a stereo nut who's also a sex fiend—someone more interested in frequency than fidelity!

HIKING

ROASTS   Naturally, her hobby is roaming up and down hills—because people are always telling her to take a hike!

He's a very religious hiker—his favorite story is the "Sermon on the Mount!"

She's such a nervous hiker that everywhere she climbs it's with mounting apprehension!

He's such a terrible hiker he's always finding himself at the end of his rope!

BOAST   I'm such a great hiker, I learned mountain climbing on a Swiss movement!

TOAST   Here's a toast to a true hiker—someone who specializes in making mountains out of molehills!

HOCKEY

ROASTS   Naturally, his hobby is hockey because he likes to keep things on ice!

She knows a lot about ice—especially if it's in a cold drink!

He learned to play hockey fast—it only took him but a few cold sittings!

She should naturally know a lot about ice hockey because she's always giving people the cold shoulder!

BOAST   I know I'm a terrific hockey player because I'm so full of puck!

TOAST   Let's lift a toast to a typical hockey player—someone who is always trying to stick it to you!

HORNS

ROASTS   Naturally, she plays the trumpet as a hobby because she's always trying to horn in on people!

He's so terrible an instrumentalist, the only kind of horn he knows anything about is a *shoe* horn!

She plays the horn so badly, she doesn't need harmony but hush money!

He's so terrible on the horn, he should either improve his execution or hasten it!

BOAST   I know I must be a terrific horn player, because people keep asking me to blow!

TOAST   Here's a toast to a typical trombonist—someone who is always letting things slide!

HORSE RACING

ROASTS   She had a great day at the race track the other day—she didn't go!

He once bet on a horse that came in so late, it had to tip-toe into the barn as to not wake up the other horses!

She once bet on a horse that went a mile and a quarter in two minutes. Too bad he didn't do so well when they took him out of his truck!

He once bet on a horse named "Lollipop" and all the other horses licked him!

BOAST   I have a great system to beat the first two races at the track—don't show up until the third!

TOAST   Let's lift a toast to a guy who never takes his wife to the track—he says there are enough nags there already!

HORSEBACK RIDING

ROASTS   I don't know why he thinks he's so good at horseback riding, because he has little stable thinking!

Naturally, her hobby is horseback riding because she rides an *oats*-mobile!

He's only a part-time horseback rider because he just rides off and on!

There's only one reason she likes to go horseback riding—to keep her troubles off her mind!

BOAST   People riding horses always remind me of clouds because they both hold the *rains*!

TOAST   Let's lift a toast to someone who really likes horseback riding because it always makes him feel better off!

HUNTING

ROASTS   You can tell he's a hunter—he's of small caliber and an immense bore!

She's such a cheap hunter she quit because she couldn't find a store that sells used bullets!

He's a very wise hunter—during the hunting season, he disguises himself as a deer!

She's so into hunting, she told her husband she was game—so he shot her!

He's a true hunter—less often missed by his wife than by other hunters!

BOAST   I'm a great hunter—especially at finding bargains at the supermarket!

TOAST   Here's a toast to a man who's a great hunter in life— he always aims to please!

I

ICE SKATING

ROASTS   Naturally, his hobby is ice skating—everything he does is rinky-dink!

She won't spend a lot of money on her hobby because she's such a cheap-skate!

Obviously, his hobby is ice skating because he's such a gay blade!

She's such a terrible ice skater, not only can she not do a figure-eight, she can't even do a one!

BOAST   I'm such a terrific skater, all you have to do is take one look at me and you can see it in my *ice*!

TOAST   Let's lift a toast to a typical ice skater—someone who always knows the hard facts!

INSECT COLLECTING

ROASTS   She's quite naturally an insect collector because she never bothers to clean her house!

Obviously, he's an insect collector because he always bugs people!

Naturally, she's an insect collector—her favorite comic book character is *Bugs* Bunny!

He came by insect collecting quite naturally because he used to plant bugs for the FBI!

BOAST   Insect collecting can have it's drawbacks—like nobody will eat my homemade raisin bread!

TOAST   Here's a toast to a typical insect collector—someone who usually starts his hobby from scratch!

J

JIGSAW PUZZLES

ROASTS   He developed a jigsaw puzzle to give people you don't like—none of the pieces fit together and the four corners are missing!

She's having the most trouble with the world's most perplexing puzzle—her husband!

He got so hungry putting together a picture of giant pizza, he ate it!

She claims putting a jigsaw puzzle together is easy—all you need is a pair of sharp scissors!

BOAST   I'm terrific at putting jigsaw puzzles together—it's finding the cardtable first that's the big problem!

TOAST   Let's lift a toast to a typical jigsaw puzzle fanatic—someone whose whole world has gone to pieces!

JOGGING

ROASTS   Naturally, his hobby is jogging—to keep his distance from the bill collectors!

She does a lot of jogging because she drinks a lot of prune juice!

Jogging is naturally a hobby for him because he's used to running up bills!

Naturally, her hobby is jogging because her husband makes her keep a running account of things!

BOAST   I have my own secret for being a great runner—just keep thinking about the great meal that awaits at home!

TOAST   Let's lift a toast to an old jogger—someone who now finds it easier to jog the mind than the body!

M

MAGIC

ROASTS   Naturally, his hobby is magic because people are always asking him to disappear!

Obviously, her hobby is magic—because she's always working on some trick!

Of course, his hobby is magic because he's always difficult to conjure with!

There's only one big thing she can't make disappear—her bills!

BOAST   I know I'm a great magician, because I can just be walking down the street and turn into a drug store!

TOAST   Let's lift a toast to someone who's great at prestidigitation—now if only he knew something about magic!

MARTIAL ARTS

ROASTS   She attracts a lot of attention wherever she wears her black belt. . . because she never wears anything else—just her black belt!

He always wears a pink belt wherever he goes—that way, nobody will dare touch him!

She had a practical reason for taking up Kung Fu—so she could order at a Chinese restaurant!

Naturally, he took up martial arts, because he's so good at chopping people!

BOAST   I had a very good reason to take up martial arts to defend myself—I was about to get married!

TOAST   Here's a toast to a hard-drinking martial arts follower—someone who is always after a good belt!

MODEL BUILDING

ROASTS   There's really only one reason why he took up model building—he likes to sniff the glue!

She may like to build models, but she's nothing like a model builder!

He wanted to build a model girl for himself but the parts were too hard to get!

She wanted to build a ship inside a bottle, but she couldn't find a bottle big enough to get herself inside!

BOAST   I'm such a great model builder, people are stealing ideas from me to build the real things!

TOAST   Let's lift a toast to a true model builder—someone who thinks babies come in a kit!

MOTORBIKING

ROASTS   You can easily tell she's experienced at motorbiking by the way she slows down as she passes a stop sign.

He's so fast on his motorcycle, he can do sixty miles an hour even if he drives only ten minutes!

She's so terrible at motorbiking, her cycle still has training wheels!

He's starting to lose control of his motorbike—because he forgot to make the payments!

BOAST   I know I'm a terrific biker—I just got an invitation to join the Hell's Angels!

TOAST   Here's a toast to a typical biker—someone driven crazy by an overindulgence in gasoline!

MOVIEGOING

ROASTS   He goes to so many movies, his doctor has warned him about creating a new disease—cancer of the eyeballs!

She's really opposed to sex and violence in the movies—especially in the lobby!

He thinks of a movie theater as a place where you can go thither and yawn!

She's so addicted to movies, she'll stare into the mirror to look at the film on her teeth!

BOAST   I like movies because they always end just as the couples are about to get married so as not to show anything brutal!

TOAST   Let's lift a toast to a true movie nut—someone who'll go to a drive-in with the opposite sex and actually watch the picture!

N

NUDISM

ROASTS   He's so dumb, he sneaked his girl out of a nudist camp to see what she looked like in a bathing suit!

She had a spat with her nudist boy friend, and now they're barely talking!

He was arrested at a nudist camp, but the police couldn't pin anything on him!

She's so dumb, she was afraid she'd be thrown out of the nudist camp for requesting dressing on her salad!

BOAST   I was the prize athlete at the nudist camp because I could run 100 yards in nothing!

TOAST   Let's lift a toast to a typical nudist—someone who has nothing to hide!

P

PAINTING

ROASTS   I hear he's a great painter—I should have him do my kitchen cabinets next spring!

She's really a great painter—sometimes she doesn't miss any of the numbers!

He thought his ex-wife was as pretty as a picture—so he hung her!

She wanted to do her mother-in-law in oil, but so far she hasn't found a vat big enough!

BOAST   I quite naturally became a painter—after my ex-wife gave me the brush!

TOAST   Let's lift a toast to a true artist—someone who can paint pictures in the nude even while wearing a smock!

PIANO

ROASTS   He's such a terrible pianist, his right hand never knows what his left hand is doing!

She claims she's great at tickling the ivories, but she should learn more about playing the piano!

I think there's something he should do with his piano—take it out in a canoe!

She's so dumb, she tied her hands behind her back so she could play piano by ear!

BOAST   I play my original compositions on the piano so fast, you can't tell what classical composers they were stolen from!

TOAST   Let's lift a toast to a finished pianist—as a pianist, he is truly finished!

PINBALL

ROASTS   She's a born pinball player—when she was delivered, her mother's stomach lit up, "Tilt!"

He's a real hustler at the game—he challenges others to pick up pinball money!

Obviously, she enjoys pinball, because she gets all her boyfriends on the rebound!

You can easily tell he's into pinball, the way he's always trying to score points with people!

BOAST   I know I'm a great pinball player, because I'm always on the ball and I always know the score!

TOAST   Here's a toast to an easy-going pinball player—someone to whom life is just one long free-play!

POLO

ROASTS   You can easily tell that polo is his game, because he likes to play the field!

Polo for her is just as bad as smoking, because she can never find a match!

He's a natural for playing polo, because he's always horsing around!

She had a special blend of coffee brewed to sip during her favorite game—polo grounds!

BOAST   I'm such a great polo player, I can even play in the rain—*water* polo!

TOAST   Let's lift a toast to a true polo buff—someone who enjoys horseplay!

POOL

ROASTS   You can tell he's a pool player—his wife always has him behind the eight-ball!

She's not a big-time pool player—she only plays for pocket money!

He likes to play pick-pocket pool—he hits the ball after you pick the pocket!

She put a game table in a backyard water tank—so she could play swimming pool!

BOAST   I don't want to brag that I'm a pool shark, but my friends call me "Jaws!"

TOAST   Here's a toast to a gal who's quite competitive at the pool table—always ready to stick it to you!

R

RACQUET BALL

ROASTS   He's such a terrible racquet ball player, he drives all his opponents up the wall!

She tells everyone she's a terrific racquet ball player, but it's only an off-the-wall statement!

They must have named his hobby after him, because every time he loses a game he makes a terrible racket!

Her husband must think she joined the Mafia because she's always talking about her racquet!

BOAST   I'm a very romantic racquet ball player because I get all my girl friends on the rebound!

TOAST   Let's lift a toast to a legal-minded racquet ball player—someone who always wants to go to court!

READING

ROASTS   I wouldn't want to imply that he does a lot of reading, but you have to show a library card to get into his house!

She's quite heavily into reading—next week she starts on the letter "R!"

He has a favorite pair of glasses for reading—they're right next to his favorite pair of glasses for drinking!

She really has a terrific library of books—now if only she could learn to read!

BOAST   As an avid reader, I like a book with a beautiful girl on the jacket—but with no jacket on the beautiful girl!

TOAST   Let's lift a toast to someone who really enjoys reading—especially if it's the will of a rich, dead uncle!

ROCK HOUNDING

ROASTS   He's so dumb, when his girl friend asked him to get a little bolder, he went and got her a little boulder!

She's so crazy about rock hounding, she took her last vacation at Pebble Beach!

He's so crazy about his hobby, his favorite kind of music is rock!

Naturally, she enjoys rock hounding, that's why she always looks so stoned!

BOAST   There's a basic reason why I really know my rocks—because I don't take everything for granite!

TOAST   Let's lift a toast to a true rock hound—someone who actually looks forward to hard times!

ROLLER SKATING

ROASTS   She bought a low-priced set of wheels because she's such a cheap skate!

He bumped into his girl friend while they were both on roller skates, and they've been going around together ever since!

Naturally, he likes roller skating—everything he does is rinky-dink!

She got tired of her old hobby, so now she's just skate bored!

BOAST   I tried to learn how to skate, but by the time I learned how to stand, I couldn't sit down!

TOAST   Here's a toast to a dedicated skater—someone who starts every morning with a breakfast roll!

S

SAILING

ROASTS   He's so terrible at sailing, he gets seasick in his bathtub!

She's such a terrible sailor, she once opened a porthole on a submarine!

He may love sailing as a hobby on the water, but he never touches the stuff on land!

You can easily tell she's a sailor, because whenever she sights a schooner she usually drinks it!

BOAST   I know I'm a great sailor, because people say I never let the grass grow under my feet!

TOAST   Let's lift a toast to a person who's a natural at sailing—someone who truly has the wind for it!

SCUBA DIVING

ROASTS   She really enjoys her hobby of scuba diving—last time she caught six scubas!

He enjoys scuba diving a lot more now—ever since he started putting cocaine in his snorkel!

Naturally, she enjoys her hobby of scuba diving—anybody can tell you she's all wet!

Obviously, his hobby is scuba diving—that's the reason he's always going around half-tanked!

BOAST   I'm such a great scuba diver, the fish have been known to take pictures of *me*!

TOAST   Here's a toast to a person who's really crazy about scuba diving—someone who wears his gear into the shower!

SCULPTING

ROASTS   He's such a terrible sculptor, when they made him they *really* threw away the mold!

Naturally, she enjoys sculpting as a hobby because she has feet of clay!

He's a terrible sculptor, because he tends to lump people together!

Naturally, she enjoys sculpting as a hobby—anybody can tell you she's a real chisler!

BOAST   I know I'm an idealistic sculptor because I put all my subjects on a pedestal!

TOAST   Let's lift a toast to a typical sculptor—an artist who doesn't cut much of a figure in modern society!

SEWING

ROASTS   Naturally, she's great at sewing—she's been needling people for years!

He may claim he enjoys his stitching hobby, but the work he does is only so-so!

She joined a sewing circle, but the women darn more husbands than they do socks!

He's a very humorous sewer, because everything he makes keeps people in stitches!

BOAST   I just bought myself a ton of steel wool—so I can knit myself a car!

TOAST   Here's a toast to someone who really enjoys knitting because it gives her hands something to do while her mouth's talking!

SHOOTING

ROASTS   He's so terrible at shooting because he's of small caliber and a big bore!

She really enjoys her hobby of skeet shooting—last time she shot six skeets!

He really enjoys his hobby of skeet shooting but he can't figure out how to cook 'em after he's shot 'em!

She has a lot of trouble while trap shooting because she can't keep her trap shut!

BOAST   I have a special secret for successful skeet shooting—
you have to sneak up on them on your hands and knees very
quietly!

TOAST   Let's lift a toast to a real square shooter—it's too bad he
can't hit any round targets!

SHUFFLEBOARD

ROASTS   She has trouble playing shuffleboard on ship because
she keeps going off the deep end!

He's a mean shuffleboard player on ship because he makes the losers
walk the plank!

She must like to play deck games with animals because she's known
to shuffle off to buffalo!

He obviously likes to play shuffleboard because he's always telling
people to shove it!

BOAST   I know I'm great at shuffleboard because I'm always
letting things slide!

TOAST   Here's a toast to a typical shuffleboard player—someone who's always willing to hit the deck!

SINGING

ROASTS   As a singer, there's one thing he gets a lot of requests
for—the sounds of silence!

She does one thing best as a soloist—singing her own praises!

He does best singing solo—singing "so low" you can't hear it!

She's a finished singer—that is, as a singer she's finished!

BOAST   My voice is so powerful, when I sing I drown out the drummer!

TOAST   Let's lift a toast to a singer really worth watching—certainly not worth listening to, but worth watching!

SKIING

ROASTS   She thought she'd like to take up skiing, but then she decided to let it slide!

He tried to learn how to ski, but by the time he learned how to stand, he couldn't sit down!

She learned all about skiing in one week—one day on skis and six days in the hospital!

Naturally, he took up skiing as a hobby because he has a two-track mind!

BOAST   I know just what to do to go skiing—have plenty of white snow and lots of Blue Cross!

TOAST   There's one thing you should never toast to a skier: break a leg!

SKIN DIVING

ROASTS   Personally, I don't see how he can stand skin diving—it must be awfully messy diving in all that wet skin!

She bought over a thousand dollars worth of skin diving gear to get back to nature—and under it!

Every time he puts on so much heavy skin diving equipment, he sinks fifty feet below the surface—on the beach!

She got all excited when she found out about the latest water hobby—she misheard and thought they said it was skinny dipping!

BOAST   I know I'm terrific at skin diving because I'm such a deep sinker!

TOAST   Let's lift a toast to a cheap skin diver—someone otherwise known as a *skin*flint!

SPELUNKERING

ROASTS   She's so dumb, she took her dentist spelunkering so he could help look for cavities!

He said he took up spelunkering because he was already at the end of his rope!

She's so dumb, she wanted to start a spelunker club for lonely hermits!

He's so dumb, he wanted his spelunker club to stage a cave-in!

BOAST   I know I'm a natural spelunker, because I like to drop in on people!

TOAST   Here's a toast to a true spelunker—someone who knows the rest of the limerick that begins, "There once was a man named Dave. . .!"

SQUARE DANCING

ROASTS   He's such an intellectual square dancer, he keeps calling it parallelogram dancing!

It's no wonder she's such a terrible square dancer—she flunked high school geometry!

His wife made him give up square dancing because he was dancing in the wrong circles!

He doesn't belong in that kind of dancing because he never does anything on the square!

BOAST   I know I'm a terrific dancer, because I always give my partner a square deal!

TOAST   Let's lift a toast to a great square dancer—someone who has never missed his calling!

STAMPS

ROASTS   Her hobby has given her a speech impediment—the glue from the stamps sticks her tongue to her teeth!

He claims stamp collecting is educational, but thinks Spain is located in South America!

She's such a dumb philatelist, she'd do much better collecting Green Stamps!

Naturally, he's a stamp collector, because he's always taking a licking!

BOAST   Many other people are also following my hobby, but I consider imitation the sincerest form of philately!

TOAST   Here's a toast to a true philatelist—someone who is dumb enough to pay more for used stamps than new ones!

SURFING

ROASTS   He attracted a lot of attention on the beach the last time he went surfing because he forgot his trunks!

She's thinking of giving up her hobby because she's surf bored!

He spends so much time surfing that some people call him a son of a beach!

She's so crazy about surfing, she decided to join the Waves!

BOAST   I'm so crazy about my hobby, I keep a full-size surfboard in my bathtub!

TOAST   Let's lift a toast to a true surfer—someone who always has sand in his hair!

SWIMMING

ROASTS   Her mother made her take up swimming as a hobby because she couldn't get her to take a bath!

He looks so terrible in a swimsuit, at the beach the tide refuses to come in!

She attracted a lot of attention when she went swimming last time because she forgot to wear a suit!

He's such a terrible swimmer, the last time he took a bath he almost drowned!

BOAST   I really enjoy my hobby of swimming, in fact, I'm almost constantly immersed in it!

TOAST   Here's a toast to a typical swimmer—someone who is a real *humid* being!

T

TABLE TENNIS

ROASTS   He's a very destructive table tennis player because he always jumps over the net to congratulate the winner!

She lost her last game of table tennis badly, because she pinged when she should have ponged!

Obviously, there's one part of playing table tennis he enjoys the most—stepping on the ball!

She may think she's a great table tennis player, but her opponents usually make all the net profits!

BOAST   I'm so great at ping pong, I can play on the table and eat dinner off it at the same time!

TOAST   Let's lift a toast to a kind table tennis player—someone who always likes to do service to other people!

TELEVISION VIEWING

ROASTS   His wife decided to put a mirror on the TV set so he could see what his family looks like!

She knows television is here to stay. . . as long as her husband keeps up the payments on the set!

He prefers watching TV to going to the movies—it's not so far to the bathroom!

She watches so many murder mysteries on TV, when she turns off the set she wipes her fingerprints from the dial!

BOAST   I find watching television very educational. Before TV, nobody knew what stomach trouble looked like!

TOAST   Here's a toast to a gal who watches so much television she has square-shaped eyeballs!

TENNIS

ROASTS   She started by playing table tennis, but she got into too many accidents jumping over the net to congratulate the winner!

He tried to give up tennis once. It was the most miserable afternoon of his life!

Her tennis game is improving—she's missing the ball much closer than she used to!

Tennis is all he ever thinks about. When he heard he was being taken to court, he brought his racquet!

BOAST   I certainly am a romantic tennis player—I enjoy winning over people with love!

TOAST   I'd like to toast a woman who could beat the World's Champion tennis player blindfolded—if the champ was wearing the blindfold!

THEATRE GOING

ROASTS   She goes to see the theatre so much, for her, every night it's curtains!

Naturally, his hobby is theatregoing, because everyone knows he likes to play around!

Her family knows she's always had the theatre in her veins—sometimes they wish she had blood!

Last night he went to the theatre for a sneak preview—after five minutes, everybody sneaked out!

BOAST   I saw a new play last night that was very refreshing— I felt like a new person when I woke up!

TOAST   Here's a toast to a typical theatregoer—someone who wants to make sure the entire audience hears his bad cough!

TRACK EVENTS

ROASTS   The only reason he made a record-standing broad jump was because somebody gave him a hot-foot!

There's only one reason she's so interested in running—so she can catch a man!

He's so dumb, he thinks to be eligible to compete in the pole vault you have to be Polish!

She's obviously into track events because she's been giving people the runaround for years!

BOAST   I'm not so interested in broad jumping as I'm interested in jumping broads!

TOAST   Let's lift a toast to a true track person—someone who is really outstanding in his field!

TRAMPOLINE

ROASTS   She's so dumb, she thinks all trampoline artists are required to have *spring* training!

He's a born trampoline artist, because he was a bouncing baby boy!

Obviously, she's a trampoline artist, because she gets all her boyfriends on the rebound!

Naturally, he's a trampoline artist, because his life has a lot of ups and downs!

BOAST   I knew it would be easy for me to master the trampoline, so I just gave it a tumble!

TOAST   Here's a toast to a true trampoline artist—someone who keeps bouncing out of bed all night!

TRAVEL

ROASTS   He's gotten so bored of traveling around the world, now he wants to go someplace else!

There's really only one reason she travels so much—to keep ahead of the bill collectors!

He likes to travel extensively, so he can come home with a lot of *brag* and baggage!

She thinks travel broadens her mind, but it only lengthens her conversation!

BOAST   My last travel trip was strictly for pleasure—I left my wife behind!

TOAST   Let's lift a toast to a true traveler—someone who goes thousands of miles to get a photo of himself by his car!

TREASURE HUNTING

ROASTS   Obviously, her hobby is treasure hunting because she already has a sunken chest!

He thought his wife was a real treasure—so he buried her!

She's so dumb, she didn't want to go treasure hunting because she heard the searchers were on strike!

Naturally, his hobby is treasure hunting, because he looks just like a pirate!

BOAST   Obviously, I enjoy treasure hunting, because I really dig what I'm doing!

TOAST   Here's a toast to a true treasure hunter—someone who works on a strictly *cache* basis!

TROPICAL FISH

ROASTS   He must be a very appreciative fish collector—his wife says he's got a lot of tanks!

She thinks her fish are all highly-educated because they come in schools!

As a fish collector, he's met the perfect girl friend—she raises worms!

She keeps her fish collection in the refrigerator—it's a can of sardines!

BOAST   Raising tropical fish is very lucrative for me because I make a lot of *net* profit!

TOAST   Let's lift a toast to a true fish fancier—someone who never orders a pizza with anchovies!

V

VIOLIN

ROASTS   Obviously, her instrument is the violin, because the way she plays it, she needs the guts!

He plays the violin so badly, people don't ask him to play "The Road to Mandalay"—they tell him to *take* it!

The only reason she took up the violin was because she thought she'd have a lot of beaus!

Naturally, he plays the violin, because everything he does seems to have strings attached!

BOAST   I don't play my instrument while making love because I don't believe in sex and *violins*!

TOAST   Here's a toast to a dedicated violinist—someone who is always up to his chin in music!

VOLLEYBALL

ROASTS   Obviously, he's an avid volleyball player, because he's only interested in *net* results!

She's written a new book about a beginning player in her favorite sport. It's called, "How Green Was My *Volley*!"

He invented a new playing tactic and named it after his favorite old-time singer, Rudy *Volley*!

She's so crazy about playing volleyball, she's always willing to go to court!

BOAST   My girl really enjoys my hobby—she's always ready to play ball with me!

TOAST   Let's lift a toast to a player who really appreciates a good volley—especially if it's off an opponent's head!

W

WATER POLO

ROASTS   She had to give up playing water polo—her horse drowned!

They made him quit playing water polo because he kept drowning the referee!

She's enjoying water polo a lot more now—ever since she filled the pool with martinis!

He created a lot of attention the last time he played water polo—he forgot to wear his trunks!

BOAST   I want to be the only guy on an all-girl water polo team—so they'll all play ball with me!

TOAST   Here's a toast to a typical water polo player—someone who hates to take a bath!

WATER SKIING

ROASTS   His feet are so big, when he water skis he doesn't need any skis!

When it comes to water sports, she has a wait and *ski* attitude!

He's such a terrible water skiier, he starts out on top but usually ends at the bottom!

She thinks water skiing is exciting, but for the person pulling her it's a drag!

BOAST   I attracted a lot of attention the last time I went water skiing—I forgot to wear my trunks!

TOAST   Let's lift a toast to a water skiier who can go over 100 yards in two seconds—over a waterfall!

WEIGHT LIFTING

ROASTS   When you see him lifting weights, it's hard to tell which one is the dumbbell!

Her weight lifting has done quite a lot for her body. Now if she could only do something about her face!

He thinks weight lifting builds great muscles, but they're all in his head!

She brings her hobby to work, too—always throwing her weight around the office!

BOAST   I enjoy my hobby of hefting up those big, heavy weights. It really gives me a lift!

TOAST   Here's a toast to a guy who started his hobby early—he worked his *weigh* through college!

WINE TASTING

ROASTS   For him, any wine dated before four o'clock in the afternoon is vintage!

She's so easy, to her, champagne is the wine of least resistance!

He's not much of an expert on wine, but his wife is a real corker!

She's an avid wine collector—so she can get a deposit back on the empty bottles!

BOAST   I really love cooking with wine, but I never seem to be able to finish making the meal!

TOAST   Let's lift a toast to a real wine expert—someone who knows a good rosé goes best with bologna sandwiches!

Y

YOGA

ROASTS   She claims she learned her yoga from an Indian, but I have my reservations about that!

He learned his yoga exercises from an Australian Indian. He's known as the Kan guru!

She makes every guest do the yoga exercise of standing on their head so she can pick up their loose change!

He says yoga exercises keep him caim, but he gets nervous trying to decide which supermarket checkout line to stand in!

BOAST   I just learned the yoga lotus position, but in order to uncross my legs I have to wait to wilt!

TOAST   Here's a toast to a yoga who's also a nudist—someone known as a yoga bare!

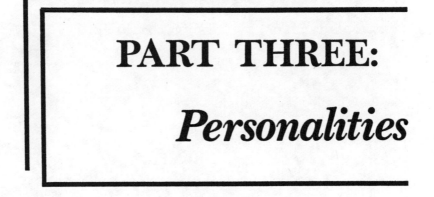

PART THREE:

Personalities

A

ARGUER

ROASTS   She argues so much, she won't even eat anything that agrees with her!

I wouldn't say he argues a lot, but his personality would certainly be improved by a good case of laryngitis!

She's great at putting two and two together—to start an argument!

You can tell he likes to argue—he has the narrowest mind and the widest mouth!

BOAST   Yes, I certainly argue a lot, but I always agree to disagree!

TOAST   Here's a toast to a person who argues so much, he should be a professional athlete—of the tongue!

B

BACHELOR

ROASTS   We all know he's a true bachelor—a man who has no children to speak of!

317

She's a girl who does exactly what she wants—she must be a bachelor!

He remains a bachelor now only because he didn't own a car when he was young!

As a single girl, she really hasn't lost anything—just think of all the PTA and Little League meetings she's missing!

BOAST   I remain an unmarried woman because I've been singularly lucky in all my love affairs!

TOAST   Here's a toast to the bachelor girl—a woman who looks, but does not leap!

BORE

ROASTS   He's such a big bore, his only shortcoming is his long staying!

I wouldn't go as far as to say she's boring, but she never goes without saying!

He's so boring, he causes unhappiness wherever he goes and happiness whenever he goes!

She's such a bore, she leaves little to your imagination and even less to your patience!

BOAST   Some people might think I'm a big bore, but they just don't realize I'm a person of high caliber!

TOAST   Let's lift a toast to a real bore—someone who not only monopolizes a conversation, he also monotonizes it!

BRAIN

ROASTS   She thinks brains are mightier than brawn, but they don't show up so well in a bathing suit!

He thinks he's got a great brain, but it's his least-used part of the human body!

She thinks she's such a brain, but she doesn't have enough smarts to make a living!

He thinks he's such a big brain, but he still can't get the lid off a pickle jar!

BOAST   I'm such a brain, I never make the same mistake once!

TOAST   Here's a toast to a real brain—someone who can turn his hand to almost anything but success!

C

CHEAPIE

ROASTS   She's so cheap she practices limbo dancing at pay toilets!

He gave his wife a thousand-dollar check for Christmas. If she's good, next year he might even sign it!

She saw a movie last week that was so bad, she had to sit through it four times to get her money's worth!

He's never been hunting because he can't find a store that sells used bullets!

BOAST   I bought a brand-new car at a bargain recently—all I had to do was file a few numbers off the engine!

TOAST   Here's to a guy who knows how to save a buck. His idea of a fun vacation is to stay home and let his mind wander!

COMIC

ROASTS   In school he was the class clown—it must have been a chore putting on that silly makeup every morning!

She may think she's a comic, but she only has nerves to steal!

He may think he's funny, but he only has a memory for old jokes that he hopes others haven't!

She may think she's funny, but her sex life is no laughing matter!

BOAST   There's really no use in my telling you my best jokes—you'd only laugh at them!

TOAST   Let's lift a toast to a typical comic—someone who proves by his jokes that the good do *not* die young!

CONCEITED

ROASTS   He may be conceited, but his opinions never change—especially those about himself!

She's so conceited, she has an alarm clock that doesn't ring—it applauds!

He always knows right away when an idea is terrific—when it's his!

She never goes outside for entertainment—it might take her mind off herself!

BOAST   I'm not at all conceited, really—although I have every right to be so!

TOAST   Here's a toast to a great egotist—a person who is truly his own best friend!

CRAB

ROASTS   There's a reason why she thinks the world is against her—it *is*!

If we took him out to a restaurant, we'd have to be sure they serve crab!

She's such a crab, she distrusts people who flatter her and dislikes those who don't!

I wouldn't want to say he's a grouch, but the reason he always feels dog tired is because he growls all day!

BOAST   I may be a crab, but I do have my way of making people happy—by staying away from them!

TOAST   Here's a toast to a real crab—the girls will verify that he has pinchers!

CYNIC

ROASTS   There's one big reason why he's a cynic, because he can't get any other job!

Obviously, she's a cynic, she thinks other people are just as bad as she is!

Obviously, he's a cynic because he'll laugh at anything just as long as it isn't funny!

She believes life is just one fool thing after another, and love is just two fool things after each other!

BOAST   I'm not a cynic because I don't believe in anything—I also want others to believe the same thing!

TOAST   Let's lift a toast to a true cynic—someone who, after catching himself cheating at solitaire, decides all men are cheats!

D

DIETER

ROASTS   He's given up eating ice cream—now his speciality is hot fudge salads!

She's on a seafood diet—as soon as she sees food, she eats it!

He's on a special new diet in which he only eats things that begin with the letter "A"—like "A" piece of pie, "A" dish of ice cream, etc.!

She eats a lot of snacks on her diet—that way she has much less of an appetite at mealtime!

BOAST   Actually, I'm a very light eater—as soon as it gets light, I eat!

TOAST   Here's a toast to a man who's always battling the bulge—to him, a diet is only wishful shrinking!

DIMWIT

ROASTS   She's do dumb, the closest she'll ever come to a brainstorm is a slight drizzle!

He's so dimwitted, if he said what he thought, he'd be speechless!

She's so stupid, she'd have to climb Mt. Everest to find a deep thought!

He's so dumb, to count to twenty he has to take his shoes off!

BOAST   I may be dimwitted, but what I lack in intelligence I make up in stupidity!

TOAST   Here's a toast to a dimwit with a soft heart—with a head to match!

DIVORCED

ROASTS   She bought real estate in Nevada so she could have grounds for divorce!

His wife divorced him because he was careless about his appearance—he didn't show up for years!

She sued for divorce because the man who once was her suitor didn't suit her!

He divorced his wife because she had a sobering effect on him—she hid the bottle!

BOAST   I may have been unhappily married, but now I'm happily unmarried!

TOAST   Let's raise a toast to a successful divorcee—she thinks alimony is a guaranteed annual wage!

DRINKER

ROASTS   Obviously, he's a heavy drinker—he's always suffering from *bottle* fatique!

Her friends were puzzled about getting her a gift—they didn't know how to wrap up a saloon!

He's such a heavy drinker, life for him is just a matter of *urps* and downs!

She started to write a drinking song, but she never got past the first two bars!

BOAST   It's true I drink a lot of suds, but I can always *beer* up under misfortune!

TOAST   Let's lift a toast to a real drinker—someone who doesn't just drown his troubles, he irrigates them!

DULLARD

ROASTS   She's so dull, she never opens her mouth unless she has nothing to say!

He's so dull, he couldn't get anyone into his fallout shelter during a nuclear attack!

Her parties are so dull and quiet, you can hear a pun drop!

He's so dull, his only interesting point is his point of departure!

BOAST   People think I'm dull, but I do have some color—my varicose veins!

TOAST   Here's a toast to a real dullard—someone who can't even entertain a thought!

H

HENPECKED

ROASTS   He's always willing to compromise with his wife—he admits he's wrong and she forgives him!

She has a very tender husband—because she always keeps him in hot water!

He claims he pulls his own weight in his marriage, but his wife throws it around!

She uses a very efficient weed-killer in their garden—her husband!

BOAST   Actually, I wear the pants in the family—it's my wife who manufactures the suit!

TOAST   Let's lift a toast to a really henpecked husband—he never knows when he's well off because he never is!

I

INTELLECTUAL

ROASTS   She thinks she's an intellectual because she can listen to the "William Tell Overture" without remembering the Lone Ranger!

He's such an intellectual, he thinks it's more blessed to be glib than to perceive!

As an intellectual, she really knows very little—but she knows it fluently!

He's such an intellectual, the smaller his ideas, the more words he uses to describe them!

BOAST   As an intellectual, I'm always willing to face the music—as long as I can call the tune!

TOAST   Here's a toast to a true intellectual—someone who always contributes more heat than light to a discussion!

L

LIAR

ROASTS   I wouldn't want to say he's a confirmed liar, because nothing he ever says is confirmed!

She not only kisses and tells—she kisses and exaggerates!

He's such a liar, he couldn't even tell the truth in a diary!

I wouldn't want to imply that she fibs, but she makes her own bed and then tries to lie out of it!

BOAST   I'm not a liar, I'm just a microscope expert because I magnify everything!

TOAST   Let's lift a toast to a liar whose conversation is like a dice game—a lot of crap!

M

MESSY

ROASTS   He's such a slob, to tell what he had for dinner all week, all you have to do is look at his tie!

The way she dresses will never go out of style—it will look just as messy year after year!

The mice are so crowded by the mess at his place, they walk around hunchbacked!

She asked the trash collector if she was too late for the garbage and he said, "No, lady, jump right in!"

BOAST   Even in the army I was untidy, in fact, I was a mess sargeant!

TOAST   Here's a toast to a messy housekeeper—someone who has his own soil conservation program!

MONEYGRABBER

ROASTS   He loves a woman for her money only up to a certain point—the decimal point!

She doesn't look for too much in a man—just a man to spend with the rest of her life!

He doesn't mind if a girl loves him and leaves him—as long as she leaves him enough!

She's not interested in any Tom, Dick or Harry—she's just out to get Jack!

BOAST   I'm just looking for a nice salad dish—a tomato with plenty of lettuce!

TOAST   Let's lift a toast to a guy with a million-dollar smile— he only smiles at girls with a million dollars!

N

NEWLYWED

ROASTS   You can easily tell he's a newlywed, because he still opens the car door for her!

She's constantly being surprised because they still think they understand each other thoroughly!

You can easily tell he's a newlywed, because he's still smiling at his mother-in-law!

She recently was married so she could have a large family. She got one—his!

BOAST   As a newlywed, I just found out mothers-in-law are a lot like seeds—you really don't need them, but they come with the tomato!

TOAST   Let's lift a toast to a newlywed—someone who's afraid of nothing, except a stack of dirty dishes!

NON-SMOKER

ROASTS   You can easily tell she's a non-smoker, because of the portable fan she carries!

He's a non-smoker, which means if you're a smoker, being around him can be dangerous to your health!

It's easy to tell she's a non-smoker—she came to a Halloween party dressed as a smoke alarm!

He doesn't have ash trays in his house, instead, he has fire extinguishers!

BOAST   I have good reason not to be a smoker—I don't want to make an ash of myself!

TOAST   Here's a toast to a typical non-smoker—someone who is absolutely matchless!

O

OPTIMIST

ROASTS   Obviously, he's an optimist—he has a poor memory and no imagination!

She's always eager to tell you to cheer up—especially when things are going *her* way!

You can easily tell he's an optimist, because he never does as well today as he expects to do tomorrow!

She always thinks that everything is for the best—and that *she* is the best!

BOAST   I always benefit as an optimist because I make the best of it when I get the worst of it!

TOAST   Let's lift a toast to a true optimist—someone who doesn't care what happens, as long as it happens to somebody else!

P

PESSIMIST

ROASTS   Obviously, she's a pessimist—she's never happy unless she's miserable!

Obviously, he's a pessimist—he looks at the world through *morose*-colored glasses!

She thinks the chief purpose of sunlight is to cast shadows!

He not only expects the worst, he makes the worst of it when it happens!

BOAST   I know I'm a pessimist, because if I had the choice of two evils, I'd take *both*!

TOAST   Here's a toast to a real pessimist—someone who feels good, for fear he'll feel worse when he feels better!

PLAYBOY/GIRL

ROASTS   Obviously, he's a real playboy—he's a man about town and a fool about women!

Obviously, she's a playgirl—she thinks life is a *fun*-way street!

He's a playboy who wouldn't look as old as he does if he wouldn't act as young as he does!

She's a playgirl whose chief interest is not the men in her life but the life in her men!

BOAST   I never kiss a girl good night because, by the time I leave her, it's always morning!

TOAST   Let's lift a toast to a playboy who can read women like a book, but he always forgets his place!

POOR

ROASTS   Her family was so poor, they couldn't afford to have her—so the neighbors had her!

You can easily tell he's poor, because he thinks more about money than the rich!

It was easy for her to find the poorhouse—it's always the last house on Easy Street!

You can easily tell how poor he is—with him, things are usually touch and go!

BOAST   I really don't mind being poor—it just deprives me of many things I'm better off without!

TOAST   Here's a toast to a really poor person—someone who's never ashamed of slumming!

Q

QUIET

ROASTS   Talk about being quiet—if silence is truly golden, this guy is a multi-billionaire!

She has a great reason for always being so quiet—she's afraid of being misquoted!

He's so quiet, they made him yell leader at the School for the Deaf!

There's one good thing about her being so quiet—she's always the *still*-life of the party!

BOAST   The reason I'm so quiet is because the person who talks the most usually has nothing to say!

TOAST   Let's lift a toast to a really quiet person—someone who's usually the one most worth listening to!

R

RICH

ROASTS   You can easily tell she's rich because she's never afraid to ask the clerk to show her something cheaper!

He's a man of untold wealth because he never reports it on his income tax return!

She's so rich, she's got bills in her wallet with pictures of presidents you never even heard of!

Everyone knows he's lousy with money—and he's lousy *without* money, too!

BOAST   I was so rich as a kid, I was the only one in town with a Cadillac tricycle!

TOAST   Here's a toast to a really rich person—someone who doesn't count his money, he measures it!

S

SEX FIEND

ROASTS   He and his wife have an ideal realtionship. She likes breakfast in bed and he likes sex on the kitchen table!

I wouldn't want to say she likes sex, but she gets her men by using *come-on* sense!

He's so sex crazy, he joined a nudist colony so he could see life in the raw!

I wouldn't want to say she likes sex, but she's gotten a job teaching it to minks!

BOAST   I'm a real expert on sex—because I always have a good grasp on the subject!

TOAST   Here's a toast to a gal who acts like she just invented sex and can't wait to spread the idea around!

SMOKER

ROASTS   She read so many bad things about smoking, she decided to give up reading!

In his house, you can't tell if the smoke is coming from his cigarettes or his wife's cooking!

She's such a heavy smoker, you can get nicotine poisoning by just kissing her hand!

He gave his wife a pocket lighter, but she'd rather light cigarettes!

BOAST   I'll have to become a chain smoker soon—I no longer can afford cigarettes!

TOAST   Let's lift a toast to a real cigarette smoker—he's always making an ash of himself!

SNOB

ROASTS   Obviously, he's a snob—he declines to be introduced to anyone he doesn't know!

You can easily tell she's a snob—she looks like she was born with her face lifted!

He's such a snob, he talks like he had begotten his own ancestors!

She's such a snob, she detests mingling with her inferiors—even though she hasn't any!

BOAST   I have a very good reason for being such a snob—I feel it's my duty to be snooty!

TOAST   Let's lift a toast to a true snob—someone who gets the wrong slant on things by looking down his nose!

SOFT TOUCH

ROASTS   She's such a soft touch, she gave a beggar three thousand dollars for a cup of coffee—so he could drink it in Brazil!

He's such a soft touch, he gave some movie producers a load of money so they could film *Webster's Unabridged Dictionary*!

She's such a soft touch, she gave the Ford Foundation a big donation because she thought it was a new kind of girdle!

He's such a soft touch, he gave his brother-in-law money for billard balls to stuff his mattress—to roll out of bed!

BOAST   I'm quite worried about the health of some of my friends to whom I've lent money—they seem to have lost their memory!

TOAST   Here's a toast to a real soft touch—he invested in low-cal shampoo for fatheads!

SPENDTHRIFT

ROASTS   He spends money so foolishly, he had stained glass put in his car windows!

She's such a spendthrift, her husband hasn't reported his credit cards stolen because the thief is spending less than she does!

He drives around town so much on spending sprees, his car has a combination safety and money belt!

She made her husband a millionaire—before that, he was a *multi*-millionaire!

BOAST   I may buy things as if there were no tomorrow, but at least I have no other extravagance!

TOAST   Let's lift a toast to a real spendthrift—someone who brings more bills into the house than a congressman!

STUBBORN

ROASTS   She's so stubborn, she's a woman of convictions—and she's served time for every one of them!

He doesn't just have a stubborn streak, he's all stubborn through and through!

She's a woman who's used to change, except when it comes to changing her mind!

He's so stubborn, he won't even eat anything that agrees with him!

BOAST   I'm not really all that stubborn—I'll agree with anyone who says I'm terrific!

TOAST   Here's a toast to someone who acts just like a mule—stubbornly backward about going forward!

T

TALKER

ROASTS   Right now, he's suffering in silence—his telephone is out of order!

Her pet parrot died of extreme frustration—it never got a chance to talk!

There's a very good reason he talks so much—his mother raised him on tongue sandwiches!

She talks so much, she doesn't just enjoy conversation, she syndicates it!

BOAST   I'm a good second story man—if you don't like my first story, I've always got a second!

TOAST   I toast a man who claims a good reason for talking so much—he was vaccinated by a phonograph needle!

TEETOTALER

ROASTS   He's such a teetotaler, he won't even accept an alcohol
rub!

Obviously, she's a teetotaler, because she's always out of spirits!

He's such a teetotaler, he refuses to have his portrait done except
in water colors!

She says she's a teetotaler, but with what she puts in it, she can get
totally drunk on her tea!

BOAST   I gave up drinking for two good reasons—my wife and
my kidneys!

TOAST   Let's lift a toast to a true teetotaler—someone for whom
water flows like wine!

TIDY

ROASTS   She's such a tidy housekeeper, her husband got up one
night for a glass of water and came back to find the bed made!

He has a sure-fire way of keeping their kitchen spotless—they eat
out!

She's such a tidy person that when she swept down the aisle, she
really swept down the aisle!

He has no trouble keeping himself tidy—he used to live in a nudist
camp!

BOAST   Sure, I'm tidy, but I just want to make sure the place is neat before the maid comes to clean up!

TOAST   Here's a toast to a really tidy person—someone who's so neat, he puts newspaper under the cuckoo clock!

V

VEGETARIAN

ROASTS   You can easily tell he's a vegetarian, because he really knows his onions!

Obviously, she's a vegetarian—all she's interested in is lots of lettuce!

Obviously, he's a vegetarian, because he's always being seen with some tomato!

She thinks the secret of health is in eating onions, but her difficulty is in keeping the secret!

BOAST   There's one great advantage to being a vegetarian—I never have a bone to pick with anyone!

TOAST   Let's lift a toast to a true vegetarian—someone who never gets to the meat of a story!

VETERAN

ROASTS   She fought with her husband all through Europe, which makes him a veteran of foreign wars!

He fought with several wartime generals, but then, he can't get along with anybody!

She's a wartime veteran, which means there's proof that the pension is mightier than the sword!

Being a soldier during the war changed nearly all his ideas—except his opinions of officers!

BOAST   I think one thing would be sure if we had World War Three—we wouldn't have to worry about any veterans' benefits!

TOAST   Here's a toast to a veteran who was a true soldier—someone to whom we owe a lot of *tanks*!

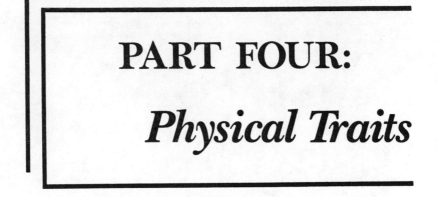

PART FOUR:

Physical Traits

B

BALD

ROASTS   He obviously believes in the old motto: hair today, gone tomorrow!

He received a comb and hairbrush for Christmas and declared, "I'll never part with this!"

He does have some virtue in being bald—he never has to part things down the middle!

As a bald-headed baby, he had a snow-white head, His mother kept powdering the wrong end!

BOAST   I don't mind being bald-headed—it only means that I came out on top!

TOAST   Let's lift a toast to a bald-headed man—with unexpected callers, all he has to do is straighten his tie!

BEARD/MOUSTACHE

ROASTS   The only thing that keeps him from being a bare-faced liar is his beard and moustache!

He has to wear a beard—with his face, he'd have to sneak up to the mirror to shave!

I'm not sure if that's a beard on his face—maybe he just swallowed a beaver!

Doesn't he have a beautiful beard, folks? His mother had one just like it!

BOAST   I grew my beard long once at a nudist colony—so I could go out for coffee!

TOAST   Here's a toast to a man familiar with an old adage— "Never spit in a man's face, unless his beard is on fire!"

BLONDE

ROASTS   She may look like a dumb blonde, but she's really a smart brunette!

She may call herself a blonde, but others say she's an outstanding contribution to chemistry!

Many people admire her beautiful, blonde upsweep—others wonder where she swept it up!

Friends asked her husband who the dopey blonde was they saw him running around with. He said, "Nobody, my wife just dyed her hair!"

BOAST   The women all call me a dizzy blond, but the men know me as a golden opportunity!

TOAST   Here's a toast to a beautiful girl—a blonde who we can say dyed by her own hands!

BUSTY

ROASTS   All you have to do is take one look at her to tell she likes to keep abreast of things!

I must say one thing about her personality, she's really an *up-front* girl!

One thing's sure about her—if she was ever in a boating accident, she wouldn't need a lifevest!

I'd like to give her a tremendous build-up, but I think it's obvious nature beat me to it!

BOAST   At Christmas, I always hang my bra over the fireplace instead of my stockings—because it holds a lot more!

TOAST   Let's lift a toast to someone who reminds me of the traffic over Kennedy Airport—well-stacked!

E

EARS

ROASTS   I wouldn't want to say he has big ears, but he's set to star in the remake of "Dumbo!"

I wouldn't want to say she has big ears, but she uses mops for cotton swabs!

He has such big ears, he went on a diet and lost five pounds just in his lobes!

She has such big ears, they'd put a Kansas cornfield to shame!

BOAST   My big ears allow me to listen to both sides of an argument—even the next door neighbor's!

TOAST   Let's lift a toast to a special man—when he says, "I'm all ears"—you can believe it!

F

FANCY DRESSER

ROASTS   His slacks are so tight, he has to carry his wallet in his mouth!

She's interested in clothes—it's too bad she's not interesting *in* them!

He may think he's a fancy dresser, but he looks like he's wearing clothes to pay off an election bet!

She has a real passion for clothes—it's too bad none can return the affection!

BOAST   My clothes are all becoming—becoming the envy of all who see them!

TOAST   Let's lift a toast to a real fancy dresser—someone who always seems to find her clothes two sizes too small!

FAT

ROASTS   She is so fat, when she sits around the house—she really sits around the house!

He is so fat, they have to run relay races around him to measure his waistline!

She is so fat, her clothes hangers are at the county airport!

He is so fat, the family hangs a white sheet on him to show their home movies!

BOAST   Yes, I may be fat, but it certainly is good of me to let you have your fun at my expanse!

TOAST   Here's a toast to a man who must be eating a lot of army food—everything he eats goes to the front!

FEET

ROASTS   I'd have some trouble naming his most dominant physical trait—because it would be quite a *feat*!

I don't want to say she has big feet, but everytime she buys a pair of shoes, the salesman gets a bonus!

Anybody who claims a foot is twelve inches long has never measured one of his feet!

Her feet are so big, when she walks in the dark, she's required to wear footlights!

BOAST   Sure, I may have big feet, but nobody else can fill my shoes!

TOAST   Let's lift a toast to someone whose shoes it would take 20 men to fill, because it took 20 cows to make them!

FLAT-CHESTED

ROASTS   She's so flat-chested, she was arrested while topless at the beach—for loitering!

She's so flat-chested, she's the only girl discovered by medical science to have *two* backs!

She's so flat-chested, her bras aren't strapless—they're *cup*less!

Her boyfriend calls her his treasure because she has a sunken chest!

BOAST   I may not have much of a chest, but I'm always the one to leave my boyfriends flat!

TOAST   Let's lift a toast to a flat-chested girl who was jilted by a real estate salesman because of unattractive frontage!

G

GLASSES

ROASTS   He's been having a lot of trouble with his glasses, lately—people keep spilling them all the time!

The only glasses she's worried about are the ones she has empty!

He doesn't really need to wear glasses—his girlfriend is a real eye-opener!

Obviously, she has to wear glasses—her entire life for her is a blur!

BOAST   Actually, I don't really need to wear glasses—everyone knows I have plenty of contacts!

TOAST   Let's lift a toast to a person who wears glasses, because he's always making a spectacle of himself!

GOOD-LOOKING

ROASTS   He may lose his good looks someday, but he'll never know they're gone!

She looks more and more beautiful—after you've had a few drinks!

Everything is good-looking about him except his bank account!

She prefers beauty to brains because most every man can see better than he can think!

BOAST   My parents thought I was such a beautiful child, they had me kidnapped so they could have my picture in the newspaper!

TOAST   Let's lift a toast to someone who attracts a lot of long looks—you have to look long to believe what you see!

H

HOMELY

ROASTS   She claims that when she was younger men used to chase her. It's funny how witch hunting went out of style!

Some people never forget a face. In his case, they're always glad to make an exception!

She looks so ugly, at Christmas, they hang her and kiss the mistle-toe!

He should only go out on Halloweeen—it's the only time he looks normal!

BOAST   I'm not as homely as some people say I am, but then, I have excellent eyesight!

TOAST   Here's a toast to a girl whose photographs do her an injustice—they look just like her!

L

LONG HAIR

ROASTS   His hair is so long, if he ever got a haircut, it would really take a load off his mind!

She used to have long hair all the way down her back—none on her head, just all the way down her back!

His long hair grows more on him than it does on you!

She likes to keep her long hair in an upsweep—everyone wonders where she sweeps it up from!

BOAST   I used to put grease on my long hair, but everything kept slipping my mind!

TOAST   Let's lift a toast to someone with stunningly long tresses—obviously, he's the *hair* apparent!

N

NOSE

ROASTS   If you take a look at her relatives, you'll see big noses usually run in her family!

His nose is so big, while walking in England he caught a cold in Spain!

I wouldn't want to say her nose is big, but for hankies she uses bed sheets!

He can't see any further than the nose on his face—but for him, that's quite a distance!

BOAST   I may have a large nose, but at least I don't keep shoving it in other people's business!

TOAST   Here's a toast to someone who has a Roman nose—it roams all over his face!

O

OLD

ROASTS   He's at an age that when a pretty girl smiles at him, he immediately looks down to see what's unzipped!

She's so old, pretty soon she'll be counting her birthdays in Roman numerals!

For him, it used to be wine, women and song. Now, it's beer, the old lady and television!

She claims she just turned thirty, but it must have been a U-turn!

BOAST   Yes, we truly do live in the age of miracles—I never seem to grow any older!

TOAST   Let's all toast a woman who really looks like a million—every year of it!

P

PLAIN DRESSER

ROASTS   He never has to worry about getting into a strip poker game—he has nothing good to lose!

Her dresses show a lot of style—if you like the style of the 1940s!

The clothes he wears will never go out of style—they look just as plain year after year!

Her choice of clothes is becoming—becoming plainer and plainer!

BOAST   I deliberately wear plain clothes, because of my glowing personality!

TOAST   Let's lift a toast to a real plain dresser—someone who's as up-to-date as a 1950 calendar!

S

SHORT

ROASTS   She's so short, she got an unusual job in the circus—being shot out of a cap pistol!

He's so short, if he ever decided to commit suicide, all he'd have to do is jump off a curb!

I wouldn't want to say she's small, but her specialty is shorthand!

I wouldn't want to say he's small, but he once had a job as a cook—taking short orders!

BOAST   There's one advantage to being so short—I have no trouble building model ships in bottles!

TOAST   Here's a toast to a really short person—someone who's all too often overlooked!

SHORT HAIR

ROASTS   His head follicles may not be cut long, but his wife had been grabbing him by the short hairs for years!

With her short coiffure, it's more hair *don't* than hairdo!

His hair is so short, he's never have to worry about being scalped in an Indian raid!

Her hair is so short, obviously she and her beautician have had a falling out!

BOAST   An advantage to short hair is that whenever I expect callers, all I have to do is straighten my tie!

TOAST   Let's lift a toast to someone with short hair—a person who's also not long on looks!

SKINNY

ROASTS   She's so skinny, she could stand under a needlepoint shower and not get wet!

He's so skinny, he got on a scale and thought it wasn't working!

She's so skinny, she swallowed an olive and was rushed to a maternity hospital!

He's so thin, he could walk through a harp without getting hurt!

BOAST   There's one advantage to being this skinny—if I turn sideways, I disappear!

TOAST   Here's a toast to a really skinny person—if he didn't have an Adam's apple, he'd have no figure at all!

T

TALL

ROASTS   He's so tall, he has to stand on a chair to brush his teeth!

She's so tall, she always has her head in the clouds!

He's obviously tall, because he looks down on so many people.

She's so tall, she hangs her laundry between telephone poles!

BOAST   I like being tall—no matter how little money I have, I never end up short!

TOAST   Let's lift a toast to a really tall person—someone who's always first to know when it rains!

TOOTHY

ROASTS   Her teeth are all her own—she just made the last payment on them recently!

I wouldn't want to say he has a lot of teeth, but last time he used an electric toothbrush, he blew every fuse in the house!

Her teeth have so much bridgework, everytime you kiss her, you have to pay a toll!

She has more teeth than a foot-long comb!

BOAST   Yes, I do have a lot of teeth, but that makes it all the easier for me to put the bite on people!

TOAST   Here's a toast to someone with a toothsome smile— while at the beach, even his teeth get sunburned!

TOUGH

ROASTS   He's so tough, he eats sardines without removing them from the cans!

She's so tough, she uses barbed wire instead of a hairnet!

He claims he's tough because of a strength-building correspondence school, but they must have forgotten to mail him the muscles!

She's so tough, everytime she sticks her tongue out, she breaks a tooth!

BOAST   I'm so tough, I keep my collar on with a nail in my back!

TOAST   Let's lift a toast to someone who's skin is so tough, they named an old TV show after it—"Rawhide!"

Y

YOUTHFUL

ROASTS   She thinks the best way to keep her youth is not to introduce him to any other girls!

He thinks the best way to recapture your youth is take the car keys away from him!

She wasted all her youth thinking about how to save her youth!

He thinks youth is the first 40 years of *his* life, but the first 20 of everyone else's!

BOAST   I believe every woman should hold onto her youth, but not while he's driving!

TOAST   Here's a toast to someone with the body of a 16-year-old—he better give it back because he's wrinkling it!

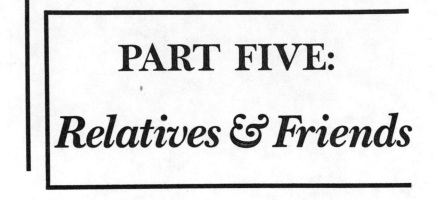

PART FIVE:

Relatives & Friends

A

AUNT

ROASTS   He knew who his aunt was when she first set eyes on him—she turned away and said, "Oh, brother!"

She's so dumb, she asked her aunt to move her piano because she heard ants can carry twice their body load!

He's so dumb, he won't take his aunt on summer outings because he heard they always ruin a picnic!

She knows her aunt would never hit her because she's *anti*-maim!

BOAST   I just bought an animal most likely to devour a relative—an anteater!

TOAST   Let's lift a toast to someone whose relative loves to work in his garden—in other words, he always has an aunt in his plants!

B

BEST FRIEND

ROASTS   His best friend is really a dear. Maybe that's why he shot him!

Her best friend still likes her, despite her own achievements!

His best friend knows everything about him, but he still likes him just the same!

Her best friend will do almost anything for her except read the books she insists upon lending her!

BOAST   I only have one best friend, because I realize that a friend in need is a pest!

TOAST   Here's a toast to someone who's truly a best friend—a person who goes around telling good things behind your back!

BOSS

ROASTS   I don't want to imply that the boss is crooked, but when he dies, they'll have to screw him into the ground!

The boss got sore when I told her I was quitting next week—she thought it was *this* week!

The only time the company has a picnic is when the boss is out of town!

Laughing at the boss's jokes may not give you a lift, but it might get you a raise!

BOAST   I may be the boss at the office, but my wife is the boss at home—she has the controls to the electric blanket!

TOAST   Let's lift a toast to a boss who, when in trouble, will never forget you—especially the next time she's in trouble!

BOY FRIEND

ROASTS   You can easily tell who her boy friend is—he's the one who reminds her when to take her birth control pills!

She doesn't just choose a boy friend, she picks him—to pieces!

You can easily recognize her boy friend—he's the one with the empty wallet!

She either demands sex equality or masculine chivalry from him—whichever best suits her need at the moment!

BOAST   I have a boy friend who's a true fatalist—he seems to pass all his days in continual expectation of the unexpected!

TOAST   Let's lift a toast to a girl who cleverly maintained her figure for her boy friend—in order to find a keeper to keep her!

BROTHER

ROASTS   Her brother always seems more interested in someone else's sister than his own!

He thinks he has a terrific brother, but then, everything with him is relative!

She thinks any of your friends can become an enemy, but a brother is one from the start!

He knew who his sibling was as soon as he first laid eyes on him because he said, "Oh, brother!"

BOAST   I asked my brother to sit on the front step because I always wanted a step brother!

TOAST   Here's a toast to a man who's glad he has a brother—otherwise, it would've been terrible wearing his sister's hand-me-downs!

BROTHER-IN-LAW

ROASTS   He didn't ask to have a brother-in-law—he just wanted to marry his sister!

She doesn't much care for her brother-in-law, but there has to be some sap in the family tree!

He took after his mother who took after her father who took after his useless brother-in-law!

She thinks if there are lazy, good-for-nothing people in the world, why must they all be brothers-in-law?

BOAST   I really have a terrific brother-in-law—he only bothers me for money every other week!

TOAST   Let's lift a toast to someone with a terrific brother-in-law—he lives in Nome, Alaska!

C

CO-WORKER

ROASTS   She has a terrific co-worker—someone who doesn't let her job take up too much of her spare time!

Who says nothing is impossible? His co-worker has been doing nothing for years!

When it comes to hard work, her co-worker will stop at nothing!

His co-worker is not afraid of hard work—in fact, he could go to sleep right beside it!

BOAST   I have a co-worker whose work fascinates him—he can sit and look at it for hours!

TOAST   Here's a toast to someone whose co-worker always makes up for getting to work late—by leaving early!

D

DAUGHTER

ROASTS   He had a hard time accepting the birth of his daughter—he thought he had a son with some of the parts missing!

When her daughter threatened to run away and get married, she made her put it in writing!

When his daughter got married, he was off in a corner crying his eyes out—the wedding was expensive!

The only way her daughter will ever have a man at her feet will be if she drops a thousand-dollar bill!

BOAST   I really have a terrific daughter—it's her choice of a husband I'm not too crazy about!

TOAST   Let's lift a toast to someone who just saved eight thousand dollars—his daughter was jilted!

F

FATHER

ROASTS   If she still thinks her father knows best, she hasn't been watching the TV situation comedies!

His father just missed being a bachelor—by an *heir!*

Her father is the head of the family, so naturally, he gets all of the headaches!

His father spent thousands of dollars on his son's education, and all he got was a quarterback!

BOAST   I must say that I'm really grateful to my father—grateful he didn't practice birth control!

TOAST   Here's a toast to someone with a terrific father—a person who became used to making allowances!

FATHER-IN-LAW

ROASTS   When he got married, his father-in-law was off in a corner crying his eyes out—the wedding was expensive!

She didn't really want a father-in-law—she just wanted to marry his son!

You can easily recognize his father-in-law—he's the one who keeps telling him, "I told you so!"

She has a very happy father-in-law—he no longer has to ask to borrow his own car!

BOAST   My father-in-law told me all about the birds and the
bees because he still doesn't know anything about girls!

TOAST   Let's lift a toast to a great father-in-law—he helped hold
the ladder when his daughter eloped!

FIANCE

ROASTS   She seems his dream come true, but she hopes that she's
not just his passing fiance!

He may look happy now, but later he'll wish he was footloose and
fiance-free!

She just had some terrible luck—her best friend ran away without
her fiance!

He's beginning to worry about his fiance—already she's starting to
whine him around her little finger!

BOAST   I really love my fiance because she's really my *altar*
ego!

TOAST   Here's a toast to a typical fiance—someone who's just
looking for trouble!

G

GIRL FRIEND

ROASTS   I'm not sure he really trusts his girl friend—everytime
they meet, he dusts her for fingerprints!

He thinks he has a terrific girl friend, because so far, their romance has been carried off without a hitch!

He doesn't have to worry about making a fool of himself—his girl friend is doing the job for him!

He hasn't been on good speaking terms with his girl friend lately—just listening terms!

BOAST   I only take my girl friend to the finest restaurants—someday I may even take her inside one!

TOAST   Let's lift a toast to a guy with a terrific girl friend—it's too bad he doesn't know she's off the pill!

GODFATHER

ROASTS   She's really got a terrific godfather—he always has a deal you can't refuse!

He doesn't know why his godfather is mad at him—he just wishes he'd remove that horse head from his bed!

She's starting to wonder about her godfather because he always makes her go out to start his car!

He's starting to wonder about his godfather because he's not even Italian!

BOAST   I'm going to get my godfather something for his birthday that he never had before—a job!

TOAST   Here's a toast to someone with a wanted godfather—he's wanted in 52 states!

GODMOTHER

ROASTS   His godmother is an always giving person—she's always giving advice!

Her godmother is a bit over-protective—she put a horse head in her boy friend's bed!

He has a very loyal godmother—she gets up early every morning to start his godfather's car!

She doesn't really know why she even has a godmother—she's not Italian!

BOAST   My godmother is really a great lady—she'd have to be to put up with my god*father*!

TOAST   Let's lift a toast to somebody with a great godmother—every time she sees him she says, "Great God!"

H

HUSBAND

ROASTS   He thought he was quite a dude before he got married—now he's subdued!

He's so henpecked, his wife makes him wash and iron his own aprons!

He's been in love with the same wonderful woman for 25 years. If his wife ever finds out about her, she'll kill him!

His marriage began as puppy love. Now, it's gone to the dogs!

BOAST   I'm really a very agreeable husband—I always agree with my wife!

TOAST   This toast is to the husband—a man who wins his wife with a lot of soft soap, then ends up washing the dishes!

K

KIDS

ROASTS   His kids are like canoes—they behave a lot better if paddled from the rear!

Her kids are so tough, they steal hubcaps from speeding cars!

His kids are such brats, he keeps pleading for them to run away from home!

Her kids really brighten up their home—they never turn off the lights!

BOAST   My kids are so smart—at age six they knew all the questions. Now after 16, they know all the answers!

TOAST   Here's a toast to a man who should really keep his kids in a refrigerator so they won't spoil!

M

MOTHER

ROASTS   He got an idea his mother wanted him to leave home early in life when she started wrapping his lunch in a roadmap!

She felt she wasn't a wanted child when her mother used to take her on long walks in the woods—and leave her there!

He was such an ugly child, even his mother said she couldn't love his face!

Her mother was very considerate—she shot her father with a bow and arrow so as not to wake the children!

BOAST   My mother didn't care who wore the pants in the family as long as there was money in the pockets!

TOAST   Let's lift a toast to someone with a typical mother—for her, the son always shines!

MOTHER-IN-LAW

ROASTS   She found the best way to get rid of her mother-in-law—divorce!

He must really be a big success—even his mother-in-law admits it!

She generously offered to donate something to the old-age home—her mother-in-law!

He recently had a blessed event at his house—his mother-in-law finally left!

BOAST   I recently got back from a pleasure trip—I took my mother-in-law to the airport!

TOAST   Here's a toast to someone who'd like to smother his mother-in-law in diamonds—but there must be a cheaper way!

S

SISTER

ROASTS   He wasn't too crazy about having an only sister—he had to wear all her old hand-me-downs!

You can easily recognize her sister—she's the one wearing her borrowed clothes!

He didn't even know he had a sister until he noticed a girl in the house wearing a nun's habit!

She thinks any of your friends can become your enemy but your sister is one from the start!

BOAST   I know my sister took to me right away because as soon as she saw me, she said, "Oh, brother!"

TOAST   Let's lift a toast to someone with a terrific sister—how about Cleopatra's brother?

SISTER-IN-LAW

ROASTS   Her sister-in-law is so mean, with her as a friend, you don't need any enemies!

There must be insanity in his family—his sister-in-law thinks she's the boss!

She didn't really want a sister-in-law—she just wanted to marry her brother!

His sister-in-law and he are a perfect pair—she's a hypochondriac and he's a pill!

BOAST   My sister-in-law hasn't nagged me all evening—she must have laryngitis!

TOAST   Here's a toast to someone whose sister-in-law treats him just like a brother—it's too bad she hates her brother!

SON

ROASTS   He's a little worried about the legitimacy of his son. The kid wants to grow up to be a milkman!

Her son likes to make the family oatmeal for breakfast. He always asks, "Do you want one lump or two?"

I'm not sure how crazy he is about his son. The last time they took a plane trip together, he asked him to go outside and play!

I wouldn't want to say her son misbehaves, but the kid always displays his *pest* manners!

BOAST   I really enjoyed raising my son. He finished both college and me at the same time!

TOAST   Here's a toast to both the honoree and his son—living proof that you can't trust the judgement of parents!

U

UNCLE

ROASTS   He'll never forget the kind uncle who helped him when he was in trouble—especially the next time he's in trouble!

She has a very sensible uncle—he never throws away his pinup calendar just because it's the end of the year!

His uncle has only three weeks to live—after that, his wife comes back from vacation!

Her uncle is a man of many convictions, because he keeps getting caught!

BOAST   My uncle still enjoys the night life—mostly wine, women and aspirin!

TOAST   Let's lift a toast to someone whose uncle is a college graduate—he can't get a decent job, either!

W

WIFE

ROASTS   He hasn't reported his wife's credit cards stolen yet—the thief is spending less with them than she did!

He should have noticed her jealousy at their wedding—she had male bridesmaids!

Her husband carries pictures of the kids, and a long-playing record of her!

He never knew what true happiness was until he married her—then it was too late!

BOAST   I've been a great housekeeper in all my marriages—whenever I get a divorce, I keep the house!

TOAST   Here's a toast to the wife—when it comes to money, her husband really has to hand it to her!